The Quadfather

Brian P. Swift

**MOTIVATION
CHAMPS**
PUBLISHING

Copyright 2019 Motivation Champs Publishing

ISBN: 978-1-7323621-7-8
ISBN: 1-7323621-7-3

The Quadfather, by Brian P. Swift
Content Editor - Monica Swift
Front Cover Design - Samantha Tunney

Manufactured in the United States of America

For information about special discounts for bulk orders or
speaking engagements, please contact
motivationchamps@gmail.com

Dedication

This book is dedicated to my wife, Monica, who has taken on so many roles in my life and done whatever it took to accomplish them with a smile on her face. This may be easy to do for a year or three, but it's been thirty years. I don't know how she does it with such love. I am blessed.

To my mom, Alice Swift, whose faith and love are unmatched. Thank you for being such an amazing example to my family and me.

To my dad, Bud Swift; the integrity and grit you have taught me are indispensable and have empowered me as a man.

Foreword

I have known Brian Swift for thirty-three years and been married to him for 30 years. I am his wife, the mother of his children, his best friend, and his caregiver. I have been by Brian's side through every trial and tribulation, delight and jubilation. Through all of this, I have witnessed him practicing what he preaches and learning how to better myself in order to deal with life in the best possible way.

As much as I have helped him physically, he has helped me to a greater degree mentally. We used to joke with each other early on in our marriage that he was the rock, and I was the wreck. No matter what the situation, he could always help me through it by helping me have an optimistic attitude and putting things into perspective. He didn't always tell me what I wanted to hear, but he did tell me what I needed to hear.

The principles of what he preaches are consistent and effective, whether they are in a keynote speech to a corporation, coaching football, mentoring, or in conversation with one of our children. You may not have the advantage of living thirty years with Brian, but you do have the straightforward wisdom of a man who has been a quadriplegic for almost 40 years. Not just any quadriplegic, but one who has achieved success in many aspects of life that include family, business, and coaching. Brian has lived a life that has been an example not just to his children but to many around him. He truly is The Quadfather.

Monica Swift

CONTENTS

1

What it Takes to be
a Quadfather

"Great men are not born great, they grow great . . ."
–Mario Puzo, The Godfather

I was raised by Irish Catholic parents on the south side of Chicago and went to a parochial grammar school and high school. My father made the rules clear; there is right, and there is wrong, and he never sugar-coated anything.

I broke my neck playing football the day after Christmas my senior year of high school in 1979. I am a C5/6 quadriplegic, and I have spent 39 years in a manual wheelchair. I would not be writing this book if I didn't have two amazing strong parents.

My faith comes from my mom. My directness comes from my father. An example of his directness arose three weeks after my accident. I was sitting in the rehabilitation institute, and my dad came up to see me. I must not have been in the best mood, but my dad said to me, "It is your job to keep you up and everyone around you up, including the family. If I ever come up here to visit you, and you're not smiling, in a bad mood, or down, I will leave."

I understood what he was saying. I understood that if I was up and in good spirits, the rest of the family would feel optimistic. It was my job to stay positive and keep moving forward—no excuses.

Now that I have been married for over 29 years and have three children, all while being a quadriplegic, I not only find myself in a position to want to share what I have done to live a successful life, but I want to make the lives of every disabled person a little easier. I am using my experience as a father and a quadriplegic and the strong traits it takes to be both to get my points across. I came across a poem titled What Makes A Dad and tweaked the end to fit my purpose. I thought it really summed up the qualities that should encompass a complete individual:

God took the strength of a mountain,

The majesty of a forest,

The warmth of a summer sun,

The calm of a quiet stream,

The generous soul of nature,

The comforting arm of a moonlit night,

The wisdom of the ages,

The power of the eagle's flight,

The joy of a morning in spring,

The faith of a saint,

The patience of eternity,

The depth of a family need,

Then God combined these qualities,

When there was nothing more to add,

He knew His masterpiece was complete,

And so, he called it …

Quadfather!

–Author Unknown

This book is written with a NO-HOLDS-BARRED approach to the issues many people with disabilities face. My advice is based on the success it had empowered me to have. It is not simple, and it is not easy, but it is straightforward.

The suggestions I give are not politically correct; they are not easy to implement, and they may come off harsh, but what is in front of you will require you to mentally and physically push yourself past anything you have done before.

Like my dad told me, "Suck it up and get it done."

I wish you the best with your health and happiness. Good luck and God bless.

2

D-Day

"Accidents don't happen to people who take
accidents as a personal insult."
–Mario Puzo, The Godfather

In my first book, UP Getting Up Is The Key To Life, I recall the events of my accident and the initial shock and fear that I experienced. I wanted to share that with you to give you a better understanding of my D-Day and the start of my life dealing with a disability.

On December 26, 1979, the sun was shining; several feet of snow covered the ground, and the wind was blowing. My deep breath was cut short by the freeze in the air. You could see your breath in the cold air. My hands were red and stinging from the chill, but there was no way I was going to put on gloves. There was nothing better than being seventeen and standing on a football field with your childhood friends the day after Christmas. We had spent countless hours together playing football, not just with each other but against each other. Today, we would be playing football together. We always felt unbeatable when we played together. There were twelve of us, and we couldn't wait to get started. We stood around bullshitting and getting caught up because some of the guys I only saw when we played football.

The teams were set, and everyone was ready to get started. The ball was kicked off, and in a blink of an eye, bodies went flying. The trash talk began, and as quickly as the game started, it came to a stop. As I ran with the football, I got hit. As I dragged the defensemen several yards, someone from behind hit me and drove me off my feet and onto the ground. It was a solid hit, but I had been hit much harder. As I tried to look up, I realized a strange warm feeling coming over me, and a jolt, a shock-like feeling, ran through me—only for a second or two.

I was not in pain; it just felt like my legs were curled up under me. I thought it was just a temporary jolt or concussion. My best friends knelt down next to me and asked me what was wrong. I asked Mitch if my legs were folded under me or twisted. He told me, "No." Then I realized I could not wipe the sweat and snow off my face. I took a deep breath and closed my eyes; everything went quiet as I tried to move my arms and legs. I took a deep breath and realized there was no pain, no movement, not even a twitch. Once again, I asked, "Are my legs curled up? Am I lying on my arms?"

Joe stood up and told me he would get my parents. As he ran off, I took a breath and closed my eyes. I was thinking, *What's wrong? Is it my back? Is it my neck? What's wrong?* I wasn't in pain, but I knew something was wrong. I kept thinking, *Get up. Get up. GET UP!* Then I started to pray.

As I lay there in the frozen mud and snow, I concentrated on moving anything—my feet, my leg, my arm. Nothing, absolutely nothing, was moving. I could not roll over; I could not look up; I could not look at my hands. Still, no pain. What in the hell was wrong? I gasped for breath; it felt like I had not taken a breath for minutes. I don't remember hearing anyone or anything.

I finally could hear voices approaching, but all I could see was the sky. I heard someone say an ambulance was called. I could hear my mom's voice, and before she got to me, I closed my eyes. Once again, I concentrated on moving something—a leg, a foot, my arm—but nothing. I could hear the voice in my head getting louder, "Move. Move. Move. MOVE! DAMN IT!!"

When I opened my eyes, my mom and dad were standing over

me. I said, "I think I broke my neck." My eyes welled up, and tears rolled down my face. All I could do was blink. They asked what happened, and I explained. Mom asked, "Did you fall on your head? Did you get hit on the head?" I explained, "No, I got hit from behind and just fell to my side. It doesn't even hurt." I could hear the ambulance approaching. I closed my eyes once again and tried to move something. I looked up at my mom and asked, "Is anything moving?" She just kept reassuring me, "Everything is going to be okay."

The ambulance had gotten to the field, and they set the stretcher next to me. They came over, and after I told them what happened, they asked me a battery of questions. What kept going through my mind was: I did not hit my head, I was not hit hard, and I was not in pain. It couldn't be that bad. As the paramedics started to position me on the board, I closed my eyes and started to pray. They were strapping me in and had sandbags on each side of my head. It seemed like it took them forever to get me on the stretcher and into the ambulance. They put an IV in one arm and monitors all over my chest. They seemed more nervous than I was, and that's when I started to panic.

I kept thinking, *When are we getting to the hospital? What happened to me?* I could feel myself taking deeper breaths. My head started to pound, and my neck started to throb, like a toothache. Once again, I closed my eyes and concentrated on moving something—a leg, a foot, my arm—but nothing. That voice in my head was getting loud again, "Move leg! Move arm! Move! MOVE!" I could see myself moving my foot, my leg, and my arms, but it was only in my mind.

By the time we stopped, all I wanted was to see a doctor to find out what the hell was wrong. By this time, my neck was throbbing, and my head felt like it was going to explode. The doors popped open, and two people grabbed the stretcher I was on. I was rushed into the hospital, surrounded by nurses and one doctor. I could hear them, but it just sounded like one voice. The nurse came in and did something to the sides of my head. I had no idea what she did, but everyone started moving. My mother leaned over and said, "Everything is going to be all right. Just keep saying your prayers"; so I did. Finally, one of the doctors came over and said, "You hurt your neck, and we need to put a halo on your head." The doctor started to explain what they had to do. A nurse shaved two spots on my head right above my ears by my temples. Then the nurse put a metal ring around my head and said, "I have to screw these into the sides of your head." I saw the half-inch-long bolts she held in her hand. I just closed my eyes.

The nurse put the screws through the metal ring and started turning them. The pain was intensifying with every turn of the screws. I swear I heard cracking, like a nut cracking. I could feel the screw going deeper into my head with every turn. I tried closing my eyes and focusing on something else, but that didn't work. They cut off my clothes as they finished screwing in the brace; then they covered me with a blanket.

I was taken to a room with more machines than you could imagine; they lined two walls. I was hooked up to numerous machines, and several IVs were put in my arm. I kept thinking, *It can't be that bad. I really didn't get hit that hard.* I couldn't believe anything so severe could have happened.

I couldn't believe an hour ago I was a carefree teenager having the time of my life, and now I was paralyzed from my head to my toes. I had no sensations, no feeling of hot or cold. I could not tell if someone was holding my hand or touching me. The only thing I could feel was the pain radiating from my neck and the bolts screwed into my head.

My parents came in, but they were only allowed to stay 10 minutes. The nurses came in every so often and checked the machines. I don't think I slept all night. It felt like it was getting more difficult to breathe. Maybe it was my nerves. I tried to convince myself that everything would be all right, and I would be back on my feet in a week or two.

Two doctors came in, asked me several questions, and started poking at my feet. I could not feel anything; I could not move anything. No matter how much I tried, no matter how much I willed my arms and legs to move, they just lay there lifeless. I started to wonder if I would ever move again. I kept telling myself I would be okay. After the doctors left, another man came in with several weights. He attached them to a rod that pulled a wire attached to the halo head brace. They were trying to stretch out the vertebrae in my neck. All I could do was lie there, staring at the ceiling. After the second night, the doctors came in with my parents. They said they were going to add to the weight pulling on my neck. If it didn't change, they would have to operate.

I had another sleepless night. I was thinking, *If I end up totally paralyzed, there are so many things I can't do, like feed or dress myself. I can't wash or brush my teeth. Can I even pee or go to the bathroom? What a nightmare!* I could feel my heart beating faster, and tears ran from my eyes, but I couldn't wipe them away. I was a very strong-willed person, and I could not afford to think that way.

I closed my eyes and concentrated on moving. My arm moved! I slid it side-to-side on the bed. I kept my eyes closed and tried to lift it, but I could not lift it off the bed. I stopped a moment and thanked God. I figured if I could move my arms a bit, I would be able to move everything in time.

My mom and dad came into the room, and I showed them how I could move my arms. My mom cried, and my dad said I would be fine and to keep it up. My mom rubbed my face, and it was very relaxing. My face and neck were the only things I had feeling in, so it felt overly sensitive. They could not stay long in intensive care; eventually, they were asked to leave. I thought, *Great, another sleepless night of staring at the ceiling.* My mind went crazy with so many thoughts. I thought of all the things I did right and all the things I had done wrong, the things I should have done and the things I could have done better. I told myself I would be a better person, a different person, when I got back on my feet. I just hoped it wasn't too late. What hurt even more was the thought of my parents; all the times I had hurt them. I was supposed to take care of them when they got older. I could not hold the tears back.

The next morning, the doctors came in with my parents. They

told me they had to operate on my neck. They were going to take a bone from my hip and place it over the break in my neck and fuse it together. They said I broke my neck at C5/6 and explained where that was. The operation was going to take place the next morning. I had a feeling it was going to be a long night. By the time my parents left, my neck was throbbing. Electric shocks were going up and down my neck like they were trapped and could not get out. My stomach even hurt. All I could do was lie there and stare at the ceiling. I could not even scream for a nurse because I could not take a breath big enough to yell.

The nurses were in early to prep me for the operation. My mom and dad were there, and so were my sisters. As they rolled me to the operating room, I figured if I did not die when I broke my neck, I would be fine during the operation. I just wanted to get it done and over so I could walk again. The operation took five hours. All I remember is waking up in the recovery room.

I didn't really come out of it until that night. I asked for my parents, but they had gone home. I was so panicked; I had no idea why. My mind went to bad places like maybe I would never walk again; I could never work, play, have a family or kids. How could I help my parents and take care of them when they got older? I would never be able to fish, hunt, play ball, or dance with a girl again. I was only 17; these are not the kind of thoughts I should be having. This fear led to anger; my eyes welled up with tears; then my body got hot. I had to get better; that's all there was to it.

After an exhausting, frightening night, it didn't help to hear from the doctors that my neck break was complete, which meant I was never going to walk again and would need an electric wheelchair. No one had any idea how much movement I would get back if any at all. I was a statistic, a C5/6 quadriplegic. This is what a C5/6 can do, according to statistics, and this is all they can do. I didn't want to hear it, and I didn't want to think about it. They took the halo off my head and put a full head and chest brace on me. I was transferred to a different room out of intensive care and put into a new bed that turned over.

It felt great getting the halo off, but pain soon set in—another night in pain lying there, staring at the ceiling. I called for a nurse and asked for pain medication. At least in this room, I had a television, and I hoped that would take my mind off the pain, but it didn't. I just wanted the night to end and the pain to go away. Lying completely still, staring at the ceiling, created a frightening place in my mind. It was like being in a black room with windows. I could see everyone and even hear them, but no one could see or hear me, and I couldn't do anything to get their attention. All I heard was my heartbeat as their voices faded.

The next morning, the nurses came in to turn me for the first time. They bolted a padded board to the top and bottom of the bed. It was tight against me. Then they did something to the bed, and it spun over, turning me on my stomach. Now I was staring at the floor and the feet of people. I was this way for about twenty minutes before they turned me back over. They turned my bed about three or four times a day. I didn't feel any different when they did this to me, but at least it broke up the monotony of staring at the ceiling.

It had been four days, and I had not eaten anything. I was going to be able to eat real food for dinner. I was looking forward to it, even though I was not hungry. I was turned again in the afternoon. The doctor came in and said that I would be moved the next day if everything went well.

My mom and dad would stand at the end of the bed, uncover my feet, and tell me to move my toes and my feet. My dad would take his hand and slap my toes and ask, "Do you feel that? Move your toes." I think he believed that if he hit them hard enough, I would feel it or move them, but I never did. It would make my legs spasm. This was just an involuntary shaking and jerking that I had no control over. I hated disappointing them, but they always stayed positive. My mom would always say, "Say your prayers. Everything is going to be all right." It wasn't "You will be all right," which was something everyone said or felt they had to say. When she said it, I felt it; I felt it in the room. Her belief and confidence were amazing.

One more night, and I hoped I would be heading to the rehabilitation institute to get back on my feet. I did not care what the statistics were or who told me I was never going to walk. I was going to the rehabilitation institute with the intention of walking. I was not going to be a burden to anyone! I wanted so many things in life, and I was going to have them.

Thoughts from the Quadfather: Now what? Accidents happen, and many lives are turned upside down and inside out. Remember, life goes on; your future is not written in stone, and you are not just a statistic. As much as you need to focus on yourself, you need to focus on those around you.

I guarantee your future rests in your ability to mentally, emotionally, and physically deal with discomfort and pain. Your ability to make the best out of your shitty circumstance will be in direct proportion to creating resources in the form of people to help support you.

You can't do it alone, so start to create your network of support and friends. Don't let the bitterness of your circumstance drive family, friends, and people away.

3

Disability 101

"Many young men started down a false path to their true destiny.
Time and fortune usually set them aright."
–Mario Puzo, The Godfather

Enduring a terrible tragedy, disability, or loss has led me to look at my life more closely and helped me understand its true meaning and purpose. We have to believe, and we must have faith and confidence that our lives are eternal and that we can live with the grace of God and have a better tomorrow.

Among the major issues a disability causes are fear, depression, anxiety, and an inner conflict because of the unknown. The person you were or planned to be may not be the person you are now because of the disability. Deep down, you may think, *It wasn't supposed to be this way. What would the real me be like if I did not have a disability?*

This occurs because your mind identifies that your life situation has been drastically changed. With the change, your disability and your mind can start to work against you. Because you can't identify with yourself as the true you any longer, self-preservation kicks in, and you start resisting change or even sabotaging future growth and happiness. Whether you are walking or riding, lives change. Your ability to accept this change and make the best of it will have a profound effect on your future.

The problem exists because your mind so strongly identifies with your abilities before your injury that it now struggles to identify with your inabilities it recognizes as failures. Your mind starts to fight you because it is afraid. This fear of failure, fear of change, fear of the unknown is common in every one of us. To move forward, you must change your thinking, which is critical for progress of any kind to occur in your life.

The change of having a disability causes us to face this fear of the unknown. Fear, depression, and anxiety can cause you to be stuck in what I call stinking thinking. This stinking thinking can paralyze your thinking from moving forward, destroy relationships, and be one of the biggest obstacles to your future happiness.

If you are born with a disability, you already know how to do and think about things the same old way because that is the way it has always been, and you don't know any different. It doesn't take much effort because it's something that's familiar. We like routine things that are familiar to us, comfortable, and non-threatening.

When you acquire a disability, the problem is, you hit a wall and may not be open to new ideas and even struggle to be optimistic. This can stop you from trying better ways of doing things that greatly shorten your path to happiness and success. New ideas, faith, and a positive attitude are often the key to success. We have to always be learning and growing if we are to be successful.

It's time to move on and get over yourself and your condition, work on releasing your old ego's attachment to who you were and old ways of doing things. Ask yourself why you are so resistant? What are you afraid of? It's time to change your thinking and think about how to move forward. There is a better tomorrow ahead of you; it will not be easy, but it's possible.

Sometimes, just acknowledging the fear that underlies insecurity is enough to release its hold on you so you can open your mind a bit wider. Make yourself practice doing small new things like reading a motivational book, exercise, or just go out and do something new.

We have been taught that failure is something to be ashamed of and should be avoided at all costs and the reality is that not everyone can win or succeed to the degree you want to. A different way may be needed to plan your life, but you want to persist until you succeed. No one thinks you are a quitter. And if that way isn't working, you will have to find a new way to move forward, a way to be happy and successful.

You need to ask a trusted friend or mentor for their advice about your situation. The reality for people, whether you're disabled or not, is that if you are not the kind of person that is appealing to others, no one will want to be around you. Are you the kind of person that people want to be around? This has nothing to do with being disabled. It has everything to do with your attitude.

What goals and desires do you have? What are you doing to work toward these goals? What are you willing to do? What kind of pain can you endure? Are you optimistic, funny, or enjoyable to be around? Ultimately, what does your resume look like? What do you bring to the table?

What is in front of you is a long journey. It will be trying, difficult, and it will break you down, guaranteed. I have been there, and so will you. The key is: not staying down. Get back up and continue your journey forward.

Thoughts from the Quadfather: *No one said life was going to be easy. I learned that circumstances could always get worse while I spent four months in the rehabilitation institute.*

I understand that every injury and every circumstance is different. I know with certainty that taking the easy way going forward will not get you the best results. You need to be optimistic and strong for yourself and those around you. This is the time for tough love, not the easy road.

Surround yourself with things that motivate you like music, movies, people and start to set aggressive daily goals for yourself. What's in front of you won't be easy, and it will take some time, but it is worth the difficult journey.

4

Expectations

"Neri was content, satisfied that he lived in a world that properly
rewarded a man who did his duty."
–Mario Puzo, The Godfather

Hope for the best and plan for the worst. I hoped that one day I
would walk, but my daily game plan was to move forward every day
with physical therapy, faith, education, and life in general. Managing
your expectations is crucial to moving forward and staying UP after
your injury. I am not inferring that you should have low or negative
expectations so that you don't disappoint yourself but reasonable
ones so that you make progress.

I don't think anyone can tell you what your expectations should
be. Not even the most experienced rehabilitation doctors, with all of
their statistics going back fifty years, have better insights into what
your expectations should be. All I can do is share with you my experiences and the experience and advice of all the disabled people
I played wheelchair sports with and peer-counseled over the years.

Even while I was at the rehabilitation institute, my hope, not my
expectation, was to walk one day. My expectations were to keep doing therapy and exercise in order to continue to get better. My long
term expectations were to finish high school, continue physical therapy, go to college, learn to drive, play wheelchair sports, strengthen
my faith, continue dating, get a job, etc.

To help manage your expectations, you may want to keep the following in mind:

- If you're expecting life to get back to the way it was, you're going to be very disappointed.
- If you're expecting life to be easy, you're going to be very disappointed.
- If you're expecting people in your life to understand what you're going through, you're going to be very disappointed.
- If you're expecting good things, but you're sitting around being depressed and don't suck it up, you're going to be very disappointed.

Unrealistic expectations can cause frustration, stress, anger, and eventually depression. When you look at a situation with two different expectations, the outcome can either be satisfying or frustrating. Let's say you are married, have two children, and you and your spouse work full time. If you expect that every day when you come home from work, there is going to be a hot meal on the table, children that are on their best behavior, a smiling spouse to greet you, and a perfectly clean house, you may have unrealistic expectations that will eventually lead to frustration. On the other hand, if you take the same set of circumstances and expect that marriage isn't always fifty-fifty, children don't always behave perfectly, things happen during the day that affect people's emotions and redirect their time, these expectations are more realistic and may not lead to satisfaction in every situation, but at least it may lead to tolerance when you come home and things are not perfect. Don't set yourself up for failure. This is why you must manage your expectations.

Your disappointments or frustration = The difference between what I EXPECT and REALITY IN THE REAL WORLD.

Since similar injuries and physical changes can fluctuate dramatically for different people with a spinal cord injury, it is important to challenge statistics and preconceived expectations of what your doctors and rehab professionals project as your likely future.

Challenging these expectations can be tremendously empowering, especially when you're told something is not possible. Don't settle for basic short-term target goals set in rehab. Create short-term, medium-term, and long-term goals and be on a mission to accomplish these, no matter what the obstacles in your way may be.

Dedicating your life during the first two to five years after injury on strengthening your mind and body increases future independence and opportunities as well. You will need to continue to exercise and keep challenging yourself your entire life. Always challenge yourself and learn about exercise programs focused both above and below your level of injury.

All injuries are unique, with no two spinal cord injuries ever being the same. Every spinal cord injury is a mystery of sort, and with intense rehab from the start, you will put yourself in the best possible position to heal and improve your life. The combination of persistence, patience, and intense physical therapy is the best formula for success.

Whatever you do, try not to let the shock of your injury overwhelm you. It may seem impossible, but with the right mindset and with time, you can find a mental state that will help you heal and one you can be content with. Keep in mind that the road to hell is filled with great intentions and expectations.

Thoughts from the Quadfather: *I am not telling you not to have big dreams or great expectations. I am telling you to move forward every day and manage your expectations. You are not a statistic! Do not judge yourself against others or what you were before your accident. You may never walk again, but that does not mean you can't have an enjoyable and rewarding life. You must move your life forward every day and plan for an amazing future. If you don't have big expectations for yourself, no one else will.*

5

It's Not Accessible

"Forgive. Forget. Life is full of misfortunes."
–Mario Puzo, The Godfather

YES, your new world will not be as accessible as you want, hope, or desire. The fact is that the disabled community that is represented by people in wheelchairs, like me, does not possess a strong presence in the world of retail outside of medical sales. It is also unreasonable to think that every building, especially older or historical ones, would be accessible.

Many older buildings cannot be retrofitted to be made accessible without adding great cost. I have seen and heard too many people with a disability whine and complain about the lack of accessibility, yet they rarely go out. Too many people are out there reposting stories of inaccessible buildings, ramps, and parking, yet doing nothing about it. Give our country a reason to become more accessible by getting out there. Get involved in your community. The more you are out in the public eye, the more people will be aware of your needs.

Get in your wheelchair and go for long rides up to a park, a store, a church, or a friend's house. If you don't drive or have an accessible vehicle, have your friends or family slide you into the front seat of their vehicle with a sliding board; then take your wheelchair apart and put in into the backseat or the trunk. Just get out and start living! Don't worry about your catheter, people's perception of you, or your wheelchair. Just go!

Just because you can purchase almost anything online these days, don't let that become a crutch for not going out. Getting out is therapeutic. The mental and physical benefits of getting out, even in our not-so-accessible country, are indispensable.

I did not drive for about four years after my accident. I will admit by this time I was getting frustrated quite often about not being able to drive. My parents realized how serious I was when they found me in our car halfway down the street, with my wheelchair in the driveway.

I took my sliding board, opened up the car door, and transferred into the car. I brought two poles with me and put them on the seat next to me. Then I put one on the brake pedal and one the gas pedal. I finally got the keys in the ignition after dropping them several times. I turned the car on and shifted the car into drive, but not before I made sure the pole was on the brake pedal.

I rolled down the driveway and turned onto the street. By the time I got to the corner, my dad pulled up alongside me. He was not mad; actually, he was laughing at me. My parents knew I was serious about driving, so within several months, I was taking driver's education.

Outdoor therapeutic recreation has been shown to reduce pain, depression, stress, and anxiety while at the same time increasing strength, endurance, flexibility, and self-esteem. Therapeutic recreation also enhances social skills, self-advocacy skills, and independence while also improving mental alertness, attention span, and problem-solving. In addition, outdoor recreation activities address what has been called "nature deficit disorder" by providing opportunities for outdoor activities and outdoor play.

Lack of outdoor play and activity has been correlated with negative psychological and physical effects, including obesity, loneliness, depression, attention problems, and greater social isolation due to reduced time with friends and family.

Today, people spend less time outside than previous generations. For example, a recent study found that children spend an average of six hours each day in front of the computer and TV but less than four minutes a day in outdoor play.

With our work, home, and play lives designed around technology that has us many times looking at a screen, this ties us not only to the indoors but many times to being stationary for hours on end. This isn't good for anyone and leads to many negative physical and mental conditions. Take advantage of the size and portability of today's technology and bring your devices outside when you can to work or play outdoors.

Get out and enjoy life. Improve your state of mental health by going to the mall, the movies, your backyard, the park, or a camping trip. Research and apply for grants that will help to pay for outdoor accessible equipment, whether that be for driving, camping, or fishing. Don't let accessibility, or lack thereof, stop you from pushing yourself, getting an education, going to therapy, driving, or even having a social life. You have real issues to focus on.

Thoughts from the Quadfather: Many buildings will not be accessible, and that will not stop you from progressing forward. I spent ten years living in a home with a bathroom that was not accessible. I washed my hair in the kitchen sink. The ramp on the front of my home looked like a ski slope, and I needed help up and down, but I never let that stop me from going outside.

My father would not let me get an electric wheelchair because he didn't want me getting lazy. We did not get an accessible van because we could not afford one, and he felt that getting in and out of a car would be better therapy and exercise. That is tough love. Lack of accessibility may slow you down, but it won't stop you if you are driven and committed.

6

It's Too Hard

"Excuses sleep with the fishes."
–Dominick Domasky

No one said life was going to be easy. Yes, being disabled is hard. It's difficult, grueling, depressing, embarrassing, and yes, it's unfair, and it sucks.

There are many things in life that are hard, difficult, grueling, depressing, embarrassing, unfair and that suck. Life and circumstances are also that way for people with or without disabilities, rich people, poor people, whites, blacks, men, and women.

Anything worthwhile is difficult and hard. It will be that way most of your life; so, in the immortal words of my father, "Suck it up." There is nothing anyone is going to say to you that will make it easier. My family and friends knew that as did my father who never budged from his just get it done demeanor.

I have never, in thirty-nine years of being in a wheelchair, told my dad or said in front of my dad that life is hard or difficult. I could not even fathom saying that to him, and I have probably only said it several times to my mom. In my dad's mind, talking about things being hard was equivalent to obsessing over it, which would only make them feel more difficult.

The truth is, when hard times hit, and the challenges you face are great, you can either let your situation define you, let it destroy you, or let it strengthen you. As I tell people I coach and mentor, "You can get better, or you can get bitter." The choice is yours to make.

Some of the most amazing, wisest, most loving, and well-rounded people you have ever met are likely those who have known misery, known defeat, or known the heartbreak of losing something or someone they loved.

They found their way out of the depths of their own depression and despair. These people have experienced many ups and downs and have gained what I call GRIT. They also have an appreciation and an understanding of life that fills them with compassion, understanding, deep loving wisdom, and tough love. People with GRIT aren't born that way; they develop slowly over the course of time. You will need GRIT to survive and thrive.

It is your responsibility to find a way to deal with this difficult time. In the end, the price of happiness is your responsibility. As soon as you stop making everyone and everything else responsible for your happiness, the happier you'll be. If you're unhappy now, it's not someone else's fault. It's about taking control of your present circumstances, thinking for yourself, and making a firm choice to choose differently. So, appreciate where you are; your friends and family are too beautiful to ignore.

So many young people seem to think all their happiness awaits them in the years ahead, while so many older people believe their best moments are behind them. Don't be either of them. Don't let the past or the future steal your present.

Life is better when you're smiling. Being positive in a negative situation is a sign of leadership, strength, and grit. You're doing it right when you have so much to cry and complain about, but you prefer to smile and appreciate your life instead. Be thankful for all the small things in your life because when you put them all together, you will see just how significant they are. At the end of the day, it's not happiness that makes us thankful but thankfulness that makes us happy.

Stay focused, confidently taking one small step at a time, knowing that the way you move a mountain is by moving one stone at a time. Every stone you move, no matter how small, is progress. What you have in front of you is a journey, not a destination.

Remember, you are not in this world to live up to the expectations of others, nor should you feel that others are here to live up to yours. Pave your own unique successful path living your life happily in your own way.

You just need to believe in yourself and what you wish to achieve. Success is what you define it to be, not what everyone else says it must be for you. You don't have to be wealthy and flashy to be successful. You don't have to be famous to be successful. You don't need to be validated by anyone else. You are already valuable.

In the midst of hard times, it's easy to look around and see a bunch of people who seem to be doing just fine. Don't be fooled by appearances. Everybody has a cross they bear. We're all struggling in our own way.

So many of us are fighting the same exact battle alongside you. We are all in this together; so, you're not alone. No matter how embarrassed or pathetic you feel about your own situation, know that there are others out there experiencing the same or worse emotions.

Not if, but when you're feeling desperate, hear me: I feel and think and struggle much like you do. I care about many of the things you care about, just in my own way. And although some people do not understand us, we understand each other. YOU are not alone!

Thoughts from the Quadfather: I am not going to lie, putting a smile on your face every day will be the most difficult thing you do. It will be even more difficult to do for thirty to fifty years, but it can be done. Life can and will be difficult. You will piss yourself because your catheter came off; you will shit yourself out in public, and life goes on. I honestly can't tell you that life became easier as time went on, but I can say that I became much stronger mentally, spiritually, and physically as time went on.

You will have to find many different ways to stay upbeat and motivated like exercise, music, and hobbies. For me, staying crazy busy exercising, reading books, hitting a heavy bag, and talking with family and friends kept me balanced for the most part.

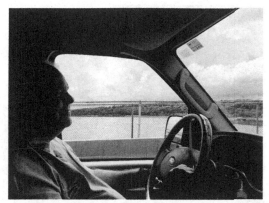

Anything is possible.

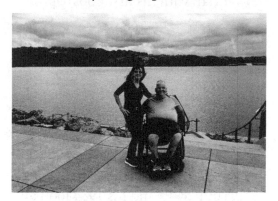

Appreciate the moment.

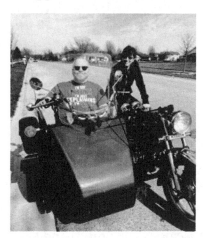

Brian and his lovely wife, Monica enjoying the open road.

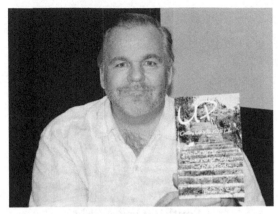

Brian with his first book Up.

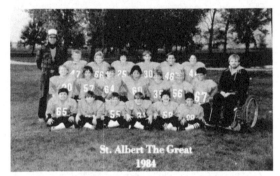

Coach Brian P Swift and his 1984 football team.

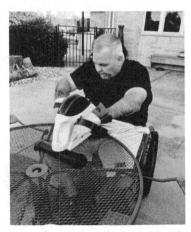

Exercise does your mind and body great.

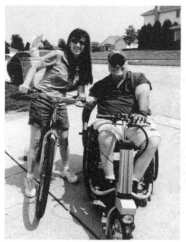

Get outside and get some
fresh air.

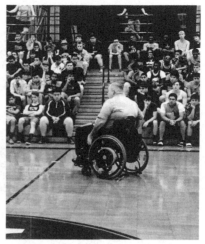

Brian sharing his message
with a local high school.

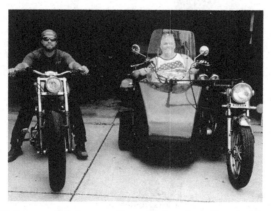

Brian and his son Spencer going for a ride.

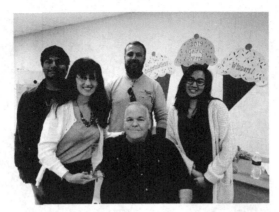

Nothing more important than family.

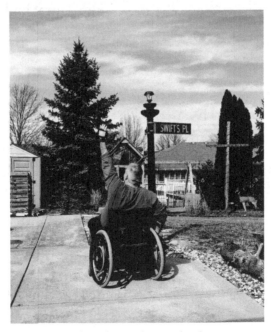

Going hard. Pushing the limits.

7

No One Understands

"Why should I be afraid now?"
–Mario Puzo, The Godfather

Yes, there are so many people inside and outside the medical community that do not understand what you are going through. Whether people understand you or not, you could spend your entire life loudly declaring to others that you don't have the time, money, energy, or resources to accomplish the things you actually want. And while all of that may be true, the harsh truth is, every single person on the planet has at least one damn good excuse for not pursuing the life they want.

The difference between the people who get what they want out of life and those who don't is that the people who get what they want ignore their excuses. They find a way around their limitations; they make a way instead of just bitching about them, and that is the very reason why they succeed.

Being disabled puts us in a position of being unique to others. Being around people with a disability makes many people feel uncomfortable and even anxious. That being said, does it really matter if someone understands you or what you're going through? Does someone understanding your struggles make your life easier or your daily struggles smoother? No, it doesn't.

People understanding your situation does not make your position or life any easier. I did not care who understood my disability, my daily struggles, my anguish, or my physical pain. I don't even think my parents, family, or close friends know these things.

You need to worry about what's important now (WIN). When you start to look too far into the future, any task or project can seem close to impossible. And so you shut down because you become overwhelmed, and you get distracted and start doing things that are comforting to you and require little thought like surfing the Internet aimlessly or watching television. That is one of the reasons why it is good to plan for the future, but then to shift your focus back to today and the present moment.

Focus on moving forward today. That is all you need to focus on; nothing else. It may sound odd, but one of the reasons the military has their men make their beds perfectly every morning is so they can start off their day with an accomplishment done to perfection. By taking the first step, you change your mental state from resistant to "Hey, I have my day off to a great start." The second reason is so when the men come back after a long, brutal, physically and mentally exhausting day, they have an impeccably made bed to come to and sleep.

Put yourself in a mental state where you become more positive and optimistic, a state where you may not be enthusiastic about taking the next step after this first one, but you are at least accepting it. Now you can take the next step and then the step after that.

In my book Rising Up, I wrote something that I would like to share with you that put me in a more positive state of mind. I kept a set of dumbbells right on the side of my bed. There was no escaping them. They were there, and I grabbed them every morning and did about fifteen minutes of lifting. I always felt like I had done something positive; so, no matter what happened next, my day started positively.

There were mornings I think I lifted while I was still sleeping. Even mornings that I felt tired, sore, or sick, I still lifted. It always made me feel better about the day and myself. Like any challenge in life, the start is extremely important. As I matured and life became more challenging, I realized I needed more than physical exercise. I also needed that faith-guided, inspired feeling I felt on Sunday. So, I also began building a better relationship and understanding of my Catholic faith and Christ.

The thing is, you can't see what the day ahead of you holds. It will shift and reveal itself along the way. That's why the best plans can fall apart, and the smallest plans turn out to be a grand scheme in your life. Occasionally, you discover that your game plan of reality doesn't look like reality.

Our lives are pulled in many directions; each one is consuming and demands time. Life is like the Olympic rings. Each colored ring represents a part of our life. The red circle is your job. The blue circle is your health. The yellow circle is your relationship. The green circle is your financial stability, and the black circle is your social life or athletics. I tell my associates, players, and colleagues that each circle connects to another circle, thereby having a direct effect on the other circles or that part of your life. You have to keep every area of your life going in a positive direction, yet focused every day on that activity or activities. I know I have to stay motivated in each area in order to make them work.

Be motivated to succeed, to improve, and to grow for its own sake. I know I personally am often motivated to do something because I enjoy the challenges or the learning experience. Every time I take on a new project, I learn more about the subject matter and about myself.

STOP WAITING for someone to understand, for someone to love you, for life to happen. HAPPINESS is achieved when you STOP WAITING for it to happen and YOU make it happen.

Thoughts from the Quadfather: To be honest, you don't need everyone to understand your circumstance; you need support. Someone understanding what you're going through does not change your circumstance.

My life changed when I stopped looking outside for motivation and inspiration. Instead, I learned to motivate and inspire myself by always learning, striving for more, always moving forward and being grateful. If you are struggling to break out, then take responsibility for motivating and inspiring yourself. Stop leaving that in the hands of others!

8

I Am in a lot of Pain

"You can't hide the thunderbolt. When it hits you,
everybody can see it."
–Mario Puzo, The Godfather

I have a broad understanding of what most quadriplegics go through, as I have been a quadriplegic for over 39 years. I also know that every injury, even if they are similar, can have very different effects. I can also talk to anyone with a disability. Yes, pain hurts, and the more you think about your pain, the worse it will get.

The first twenty-five years after my injury as a C5/6 quadriplegic, I coached football and basketball, went to school, played quad rugby, continued physical therapy, and worked in the corporate world, which meant I drove and was in and out of my van numerous times a day, all while sitting in a manual wheelchair.

During those twenty-five years and in all my dealings with quadriplegics, paraplegics, and other people with disabilities, I never or rarely heard anyone talk about pain. But in the past ten years, I have seen and heard more people talk about pain in one week than in the previous 25 years. I am puzzled by this.

I hear people with disabilities talk about posttraumatic stress disorder; are you kidding me? If that is the case, then almost everyone in the world could argue that they have posttraumatic stress disorder because of a traumatic event in their life. PTSD is real, and the effects of it are devastating, but it doesn't mean you automatically have it when you suffer an injury. Does saying that make people feel better for not stepping up to the plate? Is PTSD a pass for not getting a good education or a good job? I know for a fact that not having a good education or a job does not make your life better.

Along with more people with paralysis talking about increased pain and PTSD, they are also talking about taking more medication. This concerns me. Does almost everyone want to be on pain medication? I have talked to neurologists, specialists, and experts from major rehabilitation institutes about quadriplegics and pain. I, as well as they, understand that every injury is different. If you are a quadriplegic and have no movement below your chest area, it's usually because your sensory nerves have been damaged or severed. That is why if you accidentally stab your leg with a knife, there won't be any pain. Believe me, it has happened. That being said, and I can only speak for myself, I did not experience pain from my injury. I did have spasms that did cause some pain, but it was minimal and didn't last long. So, why are so many newly injured people with paralysis experiencing so much pain that they have to take so much pain medication?

If you have been a quadriplegic over twenty-five to thirty years and have been extremely active while in a manual wheelchair, you probably have torn elbow and shoulder tendons or have arthritis, bursitis, and tendonitis, which does cause pain. The pain I experience today is not from my injury but from overuse. Pain medication does not work very well for me due to my injury. This is when I have to start relying on other methods to reduce my pain.

Your mind is amazingly strong, and I guarantee you have not even come close to testing its limits. Your mind is able to control your body, and your mind will quit before your body does. If you have chronic pain and have gone through numerous medications and treatments that don't seem to help, the concept of mind over matter creates hope.

Chronic pain patients can reduce or eliminate their pain through different mind-over-matter methods like yoga, biofeedback, meditation, massage, or exercise. I use visualization or imagery quite often to control my chronic pain, which is in my hands, elbows, and shoulders.

I focus on the parts of my body that don't have pain and try to take that sensation and replace the ones with pain. If you can get someone to massage your neck or rub your head, bringing you good thoughts and sensations, you can empower those good feelings to overpower the pain feelings. Basically, I am splitting my senses and choosing the good feeling of being rubbed or massaged to overwhelm my pain and let it fade away. I will also listen to loud music, extremely loud; turn up the volume and reduce the pain by drowning out the thoughts of pain with emotionally charged music.

When I feel pain, I also use exercise to replace the focus on the pain and to remove or significantly reduce the pain. This is basically a diversion method, and it works. The three things I like to do, depending on the pain and the time of year and the weather conditions, are:

1. Hit a punching bag I have hanging in my garage or the one I have hanging outside.

2. Go for a long ride in my manual wheelchair. By long, I mean three to five miles.

3. Grab my ten or fifteen-pound dumbbells; go outside; and lift, lift, lift.

You know you are getting control of your ability to control pain when you can start to reduce the pain with a few deep breaths, turning on some music, or working out.

The act of dealing with your pain and getting mentally strong doesn't start in the gym. The art of getting strong starts in your mind.

Thoughts from the Quadfather: *Talking about pain is difficult because every injury is different. I can talk about quadriplegics because I am one and have been for over thirty-nine years, and I spent many years playing wheelchair sports with quads.*

I have spent over thirty-nine years in a manual wheelchair; so, yes, I am in pain. I have cramps in my legs and pains in my hands, but I have learned to deal with it without prescription medication. Understand that prescription medication is not a cure; it is a Band-Aid and not a long-term solution. Instead, I use heat packs, I stretch, I meditate and exercise when I am in pain.

The more active you are, the less pain you will be in. Pain is your enemy, and you need to fight back. The next time you're in pain, go for a two-mile ride in a manual wheelchair or punch a heavy bag until you're exhausted. Do not sit around, thinking about your pain; attack your pain with stretching or exercise.

I have always felt that if I was in pain, I might as well be productive. I worked outside the house in corporate America for over twenty years, and many of those days, I was in pain. I spent days at work pissing blood or passing kidney stones.

I would try other pain relief treatments before you get a pain pump or prescription medication. There are many natural and homeopathic remedies I would investigate, but the best way to deal with pain is between your ears.

9

It's Not Fair

"Behind every successful fortune there is a crime."
–Mario Puzo, The Godfather

Yes, what happened to you is not fair. Having a disability is not fair. Not many people in life choose the devastating challenges they are faced with. I am sure you did not choose your circumstance. No one promised that life was going to be fair. Almost everyone in life has unfair, unwanted circumstances in their lives, whether they are in a wheelchair or not. Fair or not, life goes on, so you have some choices to make. You can be a steamroller that moves forward, crushing the problems in front of you, or you can be part of the pity pavement that gets rolled over.

You may be the kindest, smartest, most interesting person in the world, but if you're not putting any of those traits to work, you're entitled to absolutely nothing in exchange for possessing them. The world owes you absolutely nothing.

Truly powerful people know that there are two basic choices: you can spend your entire life feeling sorry for yourself because you deserve more than you're getting, or you can go out into the world and actually claim what's yours. Guess which choice the more successful people tend to opt for?

Maybe the problem isn't that life is unfair; maybe it's your expectations of fairness that is the problem. No one wins all the time or even most of the time in this game of life. Unless you're winning, most of life will seem hideously unfair to you. The truth is, life is just playing by different rules.

As I have told so many people—athletes, business professionals, friends, and family—you can either get better, or you can get bitter. You need to follow the advice of author and motivational speaker Sonia Ricotti, "Accept what is, let go of what was, and have faith in what will be."

"I hate my life!" It's a phrase that's used by teenagers and adults alike. Sometimes we use it for dramatic effect, and sometimes literally. When I broke my neck, I never said that or felt that way.

Unfortunately, I heard too many people say, "I hate my life so much that I don't think it's worth living." I have seen incapacitating depression. In order to stay alive mentally and physically, you have to accept your condition and move past what you wanted your life to be and have faith that the future would take care of itself.

Here are several things I've learned so far on my journey of accepting a life that isn't fair and never will be:

When life changes, it becomes necessary to become aware that there are always more choices. They might not be the choices we want, but there are always choices. Open your mind, look around, and you'll find many more courses of action than the obvious ones in front of you.

One thing that was hard for me was being unable to do everyday tasks, take care of myself, or asking for help. I should be able to do this on my own. I don't want to bother anyone or be a bother. These were my thoughts as I beat myself up after I had to ask for help.

It occurred to me after a while that most people enjoy helping others. It makes them feel good. I know whenever someone comes to me asking for help, and if I'm able to, I feel good about myself afterward. Just think, by asking for help, you may actually be helping the other person.

I was able to grasp the fact that no one could change the fact that I was a quadriplegic. At first, it frightened me. These were professionals. They studied, worked, and knew more than I did, and they couldn't fix it.

Wait a minute …

Eventually, it was up to me to learn and use the skills I had been taught.

When my frustration rose to excruciating levels, I learned that it wasn't going to last forever; eventually, it would pass, and I just had to ride it out.

It's important to learn skills from people who have more experience with your problem, but it's up to you to put them into action. It will be scary at first doing them on your own, but the more you do it, the more confident you will become.

I was forced to make changes to my lifestyle in order to achieve and remain stabilized. Acceptance didn't make my injury go away, but it relieved a big part of my suffering, as I became aware of the steps I had to take. I have faith that I will be able to live with the unpredictability of my condition.

Acknowledge the fact that you might have to come up with another plan. Before you know it, you may find yourself thinking about the past and wondering why you didn't want it to change because your present definitely works better. Stix's song "Grand Illusion" reminds me of what life truly is. Listen to the song, and you will understand.

Life is unfair because we live in an imperfect world. Maybe some people are luckier than others, or maybe some people work harder than others. Sometimes bad things happen to good people, and other times great things happen to good people. Even if the world was perfect, fair doesn't always mean equal. The whats and whys of how life is the way it is do not matter. The key is how you deal with it.

Thoughts from the Quadfather: *No one promised life was going to be fair. Life takes a dump on a lot of people, and you're just one of them, so now what? Don't focus on fair or unfair; it is what it is.*

My dad would tell you, "If you want sympathy, it's in the dictionary between shit and syphilis." Spend your time and energy on therapy, working out, and networking to make sure you have the support you will need.

Don't think about what can happen in a year. Don't think about what can happen in a month. Just focus on the next twenty-four hours in front of you and do what you can to get closer to where you want to be.

1 0

I Don't Have Support or Help

"Never go against the family. They support you."
–Mario Puzo, The Godfather

Having to count on others to help you sucks. Yes, waiting for assistance or help of any sorts gets frustrating. Not being able to feed yourself, dress yourself, shower, or handle the remote can get you pissed off. Even more personal frustration revolves around our lack of bladder and bowel control. Combine this with no balance, no hand or finger control, and day-to-day living can become a nightmare. I wish for everyone, including myself, that we all had the means to hire someone to be our support person 24/7 and that that person could actually be strong, reliable, and trustworthy. Seeing that this isn't reality for 99.9% of us, where do we turn to get the support we need to end our misery? The first person you have to look to is yourself.

I am a believer that God helps those that help themselves. By that, I mean you need to know what your needs and challenges are and what the support is that you can give yourself. Support and help are critical, and not having either can cause distress, heartaches, and depression. Life takes care of the challenges, and it is up to you to take care of the support. This does not mean that there is no support out there. This means it is up to you to not push people away by denying help; crawling into a pity party; or losing touch with friends, family, and supporters.

It is up to you to make yourself the kind of person that others want to be around. You have something to offer others, even if it is just a smile, a kind word, or fun conversation. You are accountable for your attitude, despite what is going on with or around you.

Besides my father's directness, there was something else I learned when my father came and said this to me while I was in the rehabilitation institute. It was so important that it bears repeating. I was only in the rehabilitation institute for a month or so when my dad came up to see me. I must have been in a ho-hum mood. To be honest, I don't think there was anything wrong; I just wasn't my usual jovial self. He came up to the table I was sitting at and sat down. We talked for about five minutes before he got up. I remember him pulling his chair close to the table, looking me straight in the eyes, and saying, "It is your job to keep you up and everyone around you up, including the family. The family will go as you go. If I ever come up here, and you're not smiling, in a bad mood, or depressed, I will leave." He was not kidding.

I learned quickly that it was up to me to be the kind of person that others want to be around. I was responsible for my attitude, and it better be positive and upbeat, no matter what kind of day I was having. I was responsible to offer a smile, a kind word, or fun conversation. I decided I wanted to be that person, which wasn't difficult because I was that way before my injury. Yes, it was going to be more difficult, but I had a choice every time I woke up. I chose to be upbeat, optimistic, and a positive example for others.

If you are this type of person or become this type of person, you will have people that want to be around you. Be open to all kinds of support, from peers to family and friends. Physical support is important, but emotional support is crucial in healing from any type of injury. It doesn't matter what type of support people give you—talking, listening, or carrying you up a flight of stairs—just knowing people care and want to be with you is what helps you get through every day. I can't emphasize how incredibly important it is to keep your supporters close.

Another way to expand your support system is to join a group of people who are going through the same issues you are experiencing. If there isn't a support group for your injury in your community or nearby, today with the Internet, it is only a click away. Being able to speak with people who know your injury lingo, know exactly what you are going through, or have a way of doing something that you never thought of before is priceless. This type of support may open up your world and make you realize you are not alone.

If you think that being totally independent is the answer to your happiness, I believe you're wrong. No one is totally independent. Whether you are walking or riding in a wheelchair, you will need to rely on others for more things than you think. Being independent is also part of your mindset, the way we are all programmed to think. In life, NO one gets to the top or reaches their goal without help from someone or assistance from many other people.

Something else to consider: What does independence mean to you? Does it mean living on your own? Does it mean learning how to walk? Does it mean living without needing assistance from a family member? Does it mean getting an education so you can make money? Does it mean getting a job? Does it mean learning how to drive? Does it mean learning how to transfer without a sliding board?

I don't believe there is a right or wrong answer. I believe the answer will be different for each of us. Each of our circumstances is different, and you need to find out what works out best for you. It's not that you have to just pick out one area of your life to work on; you can choose multiple fronts to address.

I had an opportunity at the age of seventeen to go away to a college that catered to the needs of people in wheelchairs. The school was five hours away; physical therapy would continue, and I would have an aid or helper.

From the outside in, the school was a perfect fit and would service all my needs as a disabled person. It would give my mom and family a break and would definitely make me more independent. From the look of it, there was no downside, and the state would pay for almost everything. There was nothing stopping me but me. I admit I talked with my parents about all the pros and cons, and I had their full support either way I decided.

Would going away to college make me more independent? I was not sure. I could be more independent by doing more for myself around my house. By the way, my house was a raised ranch with a twenty-five foot ramp on the front that had a pitch that looked like a ski ramp. We also only had one bathroom that was not accessible.

I chose to stay at home and not to go away to school. That may not be the decision you make based on your goals and circumstance, but it was the right choice for me.

The reason I chose to stay home was that I felt I could work on more long-term fronts from home versus going away to school. I knew I would have to be more disciplined if I stayed at home.

Yes, learning to do things like get washed, brush your teeth, comb your hair, feed yourself, transfer, and drive are all very important. Support and help are critical to living a fulfilling life.

Pause and consider your life. Where are your challenges and what is the support you give yourself? You can draw from yourself the kind of support that will assist you best. You need to draw support not only to meet but also to surmount the challenges. That is how you grow.

Support plus challenges equals the best formula for growth. All of life is inviting you to grow and grow as you navigate through life. It is the resistance of supporting yourself through the challenges that creates stress, tension, fear, and unhappiness. Life is not about what you have. It's about what you do with what you have.

There is nothing more important than what is inside of you. When we develop a personal relationship with the One who created us, we discover how God wants us to respond in any given situation. By placing our faith in God, we take our hands off our problems.

Thoughts from the Quadfather: I will say with 100% certainty that I would not be as successful or happy as I am without the support of others.

Do not think that you have to be 100% independent to be successful. For the past thirty-nine years, I have needed some assistance with dressing, my bowel program, and perusing my hobbies.

Your independence will take time. You cannot be independent without an education or a job, and you are capable of both if you want them bad enough.

If you are not happy and optimistic, the people around you will not want to be around you for very long. I remember hearing this saying, and I believe it to be true, "You need to be a Friday in everyone's life, not a Monday. Remember, no one likes Mondays." You will start to turn people off and drive them away if you are not fun and happy to be around.

11

No One Will Give Me a Job

"I'm gonna make him an offer he can't refuse."
–Mario Puzo, The Godfather

Yes, it is more difficult to get a job when you have a disability, but it is not impossible. First, do you have an education that qualifies you for the kind of job you're looking for? If not, go finish school. Do you have a resume? If not, make one. Do you or can you present yourself in a professional manner? If not, learn how too.

Also, if you don't drive, learn how to or see if there is a service that will drive you to work. There are opportunities to work from home and make decent money if you have the skills. If you don't have the skills, get them. If you're on some type of assistance, and you can only make so much money, make as much as you can.

I worked in the corporate world for almost twenty years. I absolutely loved what I was doing and enjoyed the challenge. It wasn't easy; as a matter of fact, many days were quite difficult. I got in early to beat traffic and to get planning and paperwork done. When I wasn't running a training class, I was interviewing and planning.

We had sixty people hired and trained in 6 months. What an amazing accomplishment. My reward was being promoted to manage a crew of thirty sales associates. Eventually, the group got split, and I had a team of fifteen. My team put a 10% net gain on a traditional flat gain market. This put me in a great position. I wouldn't change it for anything, even though I was up at 5:00 AM and not home many days until 7:00 PM. In my first book, UP Getting Up is the Key to Life, I wrote a chapter about the ups and downs of working in corporate from the viewpoint of a quadriplegic. In the excerpt I would like to share with you now, I describe one day in particular that exposes the joys and sorrows of being in the working world.

The day had arrived, the day that cost me many sleepless hours. The day I spent years thinking about, years working hard for, years planning. I searched old notes in preparation for this massive event. What had people done well, what did people like, and equally important, what bombed? One of the biggest company events, and I would be organizing and hosting it.

I had been a part of company kick-offs in the past but never to this degree. Keeping two hundred and fifty people attentive and entertained for five hours was going to be quite a chore. I was blessed with numerous years of success, and this was a huge opportunity to showcase my other talents and abilities. I also had the gift of gab and ability to keep the kick-off fun and interesting with my slightly sarcastic sense of humor. Managing all of those corporate personalities was a trick. I learned years ago that preparation was the key. Fail to plan, plan to fail. I would not fail.

I got up at 5:00 AM and started to get ready. I always left enough time for the unexpected problem—flat tire in my wheelchair, flat cushion, catheter problems, etc. I checked out my suit several days before and had a shirt and tie picked out. The company kick-off started at 9:00 AM. It took about forty-five minutes to get downtown from where I lived in the south suburbs. I checked my briefcase for all of my notes and game plan and left. Traffic was typically bad, but I had a heavy hand. I had called the hotel where the kick-off was being held and confirmed that they had handicapped parking for a van. There it was, and no one had parked in it, which typically happened about 25% of the time.

The magical mystery tour began, getting from the parking garage to the hall where the kick-off was being held. This was like a mini-marathon, up ramps, over plush carpet that was like riding a bike in the sand while balancing my briefcase on my lap. Just a few more obstacles lay ahead of me. Ah, the wheelchair lift. It was so old it had a patina tone to it. It only took about fifteen minutes and talking to five people to find who had the keys. Oh yes, it never failed; halfway up, it stops. Of course, it goes back down, then up, yes, past the halfway point, and it stopped again. It was only about two or three inches from the top, so I decided to just jump it. There was not much room to get a start, so I adjusted the briefcase on my lap and hit it. Two big pushes, and my front tires were up, and one big push got my back tires up. There went my briefcase flying off my lap onto the ground.

I held the railing as I leaned over to try to get my briefcase. I took a few swipes at it with my hand. With absolutely no finger movement, I had to twist the briefcase around until I could slip my hand into the handle. I finally got it turned, with the handle facing me. I leaned over and tried to slide my hand through the handle. Damn! The glove that I wear to keep from getting blisters kept getting stuck on the handle. I had to sit back up and remove my glove. I grabbed the glove with my teeth and pulled it off. I wedged it between my thigh and the side of the wheelchair.

I took a deep breath and leaned over; I swung my hand, and several fingers caught the handle. I forced my hand down, and my baby finger cracked, as it got stuck on the other side of the handle. I had to slide my hand slightly out until all my fingers slid into the handle. I slowly pulled it over, then stood it up. Without having balance, I needed to lean on the top of the briefcase to push myself straight up. I took a deep breath as I reached down and slid my hand through the handle to pick up my briefcase. My hand slid right through the handle, and I lifted it and set it on my lap.

I unlocked my brakes to get going and found that my glove had fallen on the ground. I just closed my eyes and took a deep breath. Of course, it had fallen right under my footrest, so I needed to move my wheelchair. I pushed my wheelchair to the side and locked my brakes. I set the briefcase back on the floor, standing up so it would be easier to grab.

My glove was on my left side. I do not bend as well to my left as to my right, and my left-hand function is not as good. I am right-handed and do most things with my right hand. I leaned over and balanced myself by putting my head against the railing. I reached down, and two fingers slid in the glove; aha, I got it. I pulled my hand up, and the glove pulled off. My front tire was on one of the fingers.

Once again, I leaned over, picked up the briefcase, slid it several inches over, and locked my brakes. I leaned over, but because I moved over, I couldn't balance the same way. I grabbed the back of my wheelchair with my right hand and leaned over my left side. I swung my hand at the glove; it slid between two fingers, and I pulled it up.

I put the glove in my mouth, reached over, and grabbed my briefcase. I set it on my lap and put my glove back on. I unlocked my brakes and rolled to the door. I put the cuff of my glove on the top corner of the handle and pulled back the door. It opened enough to catch. I pushed my chair forward and got my knees through. I looked down at my watch, and it was already 7:50 AM. From corridor to corridor, I went as fast as I could. It felt like a marathon.

A little grin came over me as I saw the hall we were in. I rolled in, and I was the first one there. I went to the front to set my briefcase down and check out the stage. There was a ramp, a little steep, but I would make it up, and I did. I rolled over to get my briefcase, and I realized all my clothes were disheveled. I found the bathroom and went in. My tie was a mess, and my shirt was half out of my pants. I put the small part of the tie in my mouth and used my two hands to push the knot tighter. I went to pull on one of my belt loops, but I had my glove on, so I took it off. I took my thumb and slid it through one of my belt loops and pulled the waist of my pants out, which allowed me to tuck my shirt back in, at least the front and a bit of the sides. Everything looked great with my suit jacket back on.

I re-entered the hall as other guests were arriving. We had numerous presenters who all, of course, asked for a change in the agenda. I had requested several microphones because I needed one, and we needed one for the presenters at the podium. I tested them out, and we were ready to go. The hall started filling up at that time. I tried not to drink too much because I didn't want to have to use the bathroom during the kick-off.

I spent the next twenty minutes meeting and greeting people and answering questions. I took little sips of water so my mouth would not dry out. I prepared my notes and made sure the room was ready to go. The kick-off started, and everything was going great. Introductions went well, the jokes were a big hit, and we were off to a great start. The presentations were all on schedule, and I was getting a lot of good feedback during the break.

During the break, I realized my leg bag was full. Shit! I hadn't even been drinking. I didn't think I was urinating that much, but it was full, and it needed to be emptied. There was no way I could wait an hour or longer. I would be wet from head to toe. I headed to the doors, trying not to make eye contact with anyone, or I might have to stop and talk. That was not the bad part. The bad part was, I only had five minutes at best.

Of course, the bathroom was about thirty yards from where I was. I raced down to the bathroom and busted in the door. A gasp of air came out of me when I saw feet on the floor of the only handicapped stall. I looked at my watch, looked back at the stall, and grimaced. I was sitting there, thinking, *Come on, come on, come on. Just wait until this meathead comes out!* I heard the door unlock, and I spun around, just waiting to say something less than pleasant. The door opened up as I rolled closer, and the vice president walked out.

I put a grin on my face and smiled. You could tell he felt awkward and gave me the "When you've got to go, you got to go" look. I rushed in because I had to go. It was a small stall. I took my glove off and put it on my lap. I had to reach under my knee and throw my foot over the edge of the toilet seat so I could empty my leg bag. As I lifted my leg up, my foot hit the side of the toilet and didn't get near the top. I took a deep breath, unlocked my chair, and moved my wheelchair back to give my leg a little more room to swing to get my foot on the top of the seat. I pulled my leg up and swung it, but it hit the side of the toilet because I did not lift it high enough. The suit pants I had on fit a little differently than my other pants, and it was making it difficult to swing my leg up. I took a deep breath, grabbed under my leg, pulled back, and swung my leg. Finally, my ankle landed on the top of the toilet seat!

I took a look at my watch and almost started to panic. I reached down and pulled my pant leg up by using the knuckles on both hands to grab the side of my pants by my knee and yanked up. My pant leg came up enough so I could slide my sock down and grab the clamp and tube to empty my leg bag. Damn, my socks were pulled up high, and great, they were a new pair, so they were very tight, making it hard to get my tube out. I grabbed the tube and yanked it out. All I had to do was open the clamp by forcing my thumb under the end of the clamp, flicking my hand, forcing my thumb up, and unclamping it. I got my thumb under the end of the clamp, flicked my wrist, and POP, it opened, and SPLASH, the clamp came off the tube and hit the water in the toilet.

I thought, *Come on! You have got to be shitting me!* I unlocked my wheelchair and pushed my chair closer to the toilet so I could reach in and try to grab the tube and clamp that had come off the bag. I lunged forward and thrust my hand in the toilet. The tube got wedged between my fingers, and I got it out on my first try. Then I needed to try to get it back on, or nothing would stop the urine from running out the bottom of my leg bag.

I was waiting for someone to come in, looking for me. I could mentally see the door flying open, and someone screaming my name. I didn't know what I would say. It seemed like I was in there for twenty minutes. I could just imagine getting back to the hall and seeing the president up at the podium.

I pulled my pant leg up and put the tube and clamp between my thumbs. I leaned forward and lined up the end of the tube with the end of the bag and pulled it over the end. I got the tube to stick on, so I reached back down and shimmed it on a little bit more. That was the only thing that went right. All I had to do was pull my leg off the toilet seat and get back to the kick-off.

I reached down, grabbed under my knee with my right hand, and threw my left hand behind the handle of my wheelchair for balance. I pulled up, and it looked like my foot was going to come off in one try. As my shoe and foot were coming over the edge, my heel caught the rim of the lid and pulled my shoe off. SPLASH! My shoe fell in the toilet. My foot came out, but I needed to retrieve my shoe from the toilet. I unlocked my brakes and moved up to grab my shoe. I reached in the toilet and stuck my hand in the shoe and grabbed it. I held it to the side and let it drip off as I figured out how to get it on.

I lifted the shoe to my mouth and pulled the ends of the laces with my teeth. I opened the shoe up. I unlocked my chair and faced the wall. I got about three inches from the wall so I could lean over and try to drop the shoe on my footrest, lift my foot, and try to slide it in. I grabbed my shoe, leaned over, and dropped it. It landed right on the footrest. I lifted my leg by grabbing under my knee and lifting up. I tried to get my toes in my shoe and pushed down on my knee to force my foot in. After several tries, my foot would not go in, so I decided to leave it the way it was and head back, hoping no one would notice.

I raced out of the stall, slid my hand under the handle on the door, and pulled it open. I raced down the hall, trying to catch my breath. It was nice to see people milling around outside the hall. I took a deep breath and tucked in my shirt, fixed my tie, then went in. I raced up the ramp and grabbed my notes. Before looking at them, I asked everyone to take their seats.

No one had noticed my foot halfway out of my shoe, and no one had commented on the long break. I had to get things moving and get our next presenter up in order to stay on schedule. As everyone settled in, I looked at my notes, and something seemed wrong. I had looked at my notes and the agenda so many times that I knew something was askew.

As I looked into the audience, I saw some familiar faces looking back and grinning. Not in an "I am happy to be here" or "I am having fun" way. It was that "Did you notice how we added verbiage and rearranged the order of your notes while you were gone?" kind of smirk. All I could do was nod my head and smile back. Thank God I had gone over the agenda so many times that I knew it by heart.

Besides that, this was nothing compared to my bathroom ordeal. The thing my friends and associates forgot was that I had a microphone, and that was a dangerous thing, especially when I asked everyone to say a silent prayer that Tom's surgery for getting snipped would go well. I reassured them he would be fine because he was going to an excellent micro-surgeon who was experienced in working under a microscope.

There is nothing better than the roar of a crowd. I had to glance at all the executives to see their reactions, and they were all good. The next speaker was introduced, and the kick-off went on without any flaws. We had a quick break near the end, and I was fortunate to have several good friends close by, one of whom I asked to slip my foot in my shoe and tie it. Ah, one less thing to worry about.

The kick-off ended, and I was relieved. The event was a success, and I was flawless. It was a great night standing around, relaxing, having a few drinks. That was a big moment in my career. People decided to go to a piano bar to hang out, so we all headed out. I grabbed my briefcase, put it on my lap, and headed to my van. It was a long day, and I was dragging, but it was a great day.

I was leery heading back to my van as I approached the dreaded lift. Thank God it worked. Lifts seem to always work when you're going down, and this one did. I went down the hall and into the garage that had smooth concrete, which made it much easier to push my chair. I turned around the corner to my van, and SHIT, someone had parked next to me on the side my ramp was on, so I could not get in.

I looked around to see if I could find someone to pull my van out a bit. I rolled through the parking garage, looking for anyone. I couldn't believe there was no one around. I knew it was late, but there were plenty of cars there. I finally saw a man walking, and I asked him if he could pull my van out. He was helpful and did so. I quickly transferred to my seat, and I was off. I found the piano bar, but parking with a van made it a little challenging. I had to park about six blocks away. I rolled up my sleeves and headed down the road. The city was far from accessible, so I had to ride on the street most of the way there. I thought the ride back to my van that evening was going to be interesting.

I did not embellish the retelling of this event. Everything that I said actually happened to me. Believe it or not, that was not a one-time event. This type of crazy event happens quite regularly, sometimes just to me, sometimes to Monica and me. I have learned to take a deep breath and smile. I have learned to try to turn circumstance into opportunities.

Some of the people that have read that part of my first book have told me that they would never be able to work under those conditions. They are the shortsighted people who only see the negative side of things. I love hearing from the people who have read that and tell me after they read that they realized anything is possible.

Not all days at work were that good, and not all days were that bad. The point is, I went out there and found a wonderful, hard, demanding, rewarding job and didn't let my disability get in the way. The years I spent working in corporate were some of the best years of my life!

Thoughts from the Quadfather: Getting a job is within your control, especially with today's technology. This has opened up a large market for people to work from home.

Get a degree if you don't have one. The government may possibly pay for most of it. Research grants for educating the disabled. When you go for an interview, dress and make sure you look like anyone else in that business. Put on a shirt and tie if it's that type of business. You are selling yourself. Act like you will be an asset to that company.

I broke my neck when I was seventeen. I am a C5/6 quad. I finished high school and started junior college that summer and received my associate's degree in two years. Two years later, I got my bachelor's degree. Through all four years, I did not drive on my own.

Just continue to move forward, and a job will be there, even if it means starting your own business.

12

I Can't Drive

"What drives you and what moves you are two different things."
–Brian P. Swift, The Quadfather

Yes, not driving sucks and limits your options for being independent. Yes, driving will open up your world and create independence for you, but don't use it as an excuse for not moving forward. I went to four years of college and three years of law school riding an accessible bus or occasionally jamming myself into the front seat of a friend's car. I went out socially and dated before I started driving, so don't let this stop you from the big things like school, therapy, exercise, or even work.

Getting back driving will come, but you must be patient because driving takes a lot of strength, and it is very expensive to retrofit a vehicle with adaptive controls. So, if you want to drive, you have a lot of work to do.

First, if you're a C5 or lower, meaning C6, C7, or T, you need to be spending most of your day in a manual wheelchair. I have seen a trend in the past fifteen years, and that is to quickly get any SCI person in an electric wheelchair. Why? Because it makes life easier, but easier does not always mean better. Pushing a manual wheelchair is great exercise. Don't concede to an electric wheelchair too quickly.

Second, start looking for grants and funding because driving is an expensive endeavor. Unfortunately, your insurance most likely will not pay for your vehicle modifications because, according to the insurance company, they are not a medical necessity. There are numerous non-profit companies that offer grant opportunities. Just google grants for people with spinal cord injuries. I also recommend starting some kind of crowdfunding—for example, start a GoFund-Me page.

I went four years before I started driving again. When I wanted to socialize, I invited friends over to my house or went over to my friends' houses—those who lived in the neighborhood. As for going out, my friends would just lift me into the front seat of a car and throw my wheelchair in the trunk. This was in a time when my wheelchair weighed sixty pounds and did not come apart like the wheelchairs do today.

When I first started driving, it was in an old two-door car, with the back seat removed so the wheelchair could go there. I could get myself into the car using a sliding board, but I needed help with the wheelchair.

I drove a car for four years before I got my first van. Driving a van would give me even more freedom to come and go. I spent about a year doing some fundraising to help with the expenses. I also chose to drive from the captain's chair that came with the van rather than driving from my wheelchair. I recommend this for several reasons. First, it is a great way to get exercise. Transferring over allows you to work on your balance and strength. More importantly, it is relieving pressure from your backside, which is critical to prevent pressure sores. Secondly, it feels great getting out of your wheelchair and sitting in a comfortable seat. Once again, it's not easy some days, but it's good for you.

Being disabled is expensive. It is a difficult, grueling, sometimes depressing full-time job dealing with many greedy transportation equipment companies that are middlemen for the manufactures of accessible transportation equipment. It used to be different. Many companies would let you go out and buy your own vehicle and just put on the needed accessible equipment onto your vehicle to enable you to drive it. Now, companies want you to buy the already adapted vehicles from them, and they charge astronomical prices and act like they are doing you a favor for even allowing you to drive. About ten years ago, the government put into effect some restrictions and requirements for adaptive equipment in vehicles due to lawsuits. These restrictions and requirements in no way benefit the disabled driver. Once again, this is an example of us having to pay for other people's 'sins.'

The entire process can be very frustrating, but don't give up. There are some very kind, honest, and caring people in the industry who still want to help others.

So, strap it on and suck it up; you're in for an interesting ride.

Thoughts from the Quadfather: *You can find reasonably priced used vans or cars on several web sites like http://disableddealer.com. I did not drive until four years after my accident, and I was able to finish high school and college. You don't have to drive to be happy or productive.*

13

I Don't Believe Things Will Get Better

"Among reasonable men problems of business
could always be solved."
–Mario Puzo, The Godfather

None of us knows what the future will bring. You're most likely not a psychic, so stop worrying about things no one can predict. It is just a bullshit excuse for not moving forward. Whether you're walking, limping, crawling, or confined to a wheelchair, no one knows with any certainty the changes that could happen.

You can sit indoors all day, conceptualizing a better world, but until you get out there and start implementing change, you're not actually making a difference. Good intention is a wonderful thing, but unless it's coupled with action, it counts for nothing. The road to hell is paved with good intentions. At the end of the day, your character is determined by what you do, not by what you think about doing.

Every one of us has good days and bad days. Every person has problems and sorrows; some you can see, some you can't. We're not perfect, and we'll never be. It's important to remember the fact that sometimes we go through good times, sometimes we go through bad times. When the bad times arrive, be prepared because tough times don't last, but tough people do.

You need to think about What's Important Now (WIN). What's your alternative plan? Waiting to see if you walk or get stronger is a shitty way to approach your situation and your life. Assume you're not going to walk, but never give up hope. Your circumstance has not changed. What's Important Now: therapy or continuous rehabbing, getting more education if needed, getting a job, creating a network of friends and helpers.

Another way to change your beliefs and your attitude is to stop the stinking thinking and spend some time thinking of others. Stinking thinking happens when you spend too much time listening to the negative voice in your head. Controlling your self-talk is really critical to your future. I bet that you're always allowing your other voice to take over your mind, and it often gets you in trouble. Unfortunately, most of our self-talk is negative. Start making a distinction between the two voices and stop allowing the stinking thinking, big-mouthed monster in your brain take the control again.

When you're good to others, you get a feeling that you were sent on earth with a purpose. Having a sense of purpose is extremely healing for people. You can create a sense of purpose by doing and thinking of others. When another human being honestly thanks you for your kind deeds, your heart gets filled with joy.

Yes, you can keep on going by adding in learning how to drive, learning how to transfer, playing sports, or getting back outdoors. You have plenty to focus on to keep you busy. You should also reward yourself from time to time. Go out, do something you enjoy, buy something that you've always wanted. The feeling of reward is often helpful for cultivating an optimistic attitude and belief system.

Who says you can't be happy? Who says you can't do what you want to do? You can always change the way you perceive the world. You can find new meanings and purposes, and you can live your life intensively and happily. No one is supposed to spend his or her life in fear, disappointment, and unhappiness. It's your choice. Stop identifying yourself as disabled and go attack a happy life.

Thoughts from the Quadfather: *No one can predict the future. What you believe is extremely important and critical to your future* *happiness and success. It doesn't matter what the doctors, statistics, therapist, or others think because your attitude and belief that there is a better future will drive you and the people around you. I am not suggesting you will ever walk again, but you don't need to walk to have a good life. You alone have the responsibility to shape your life.*

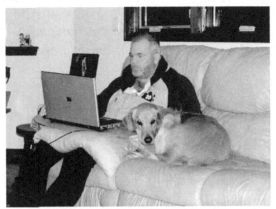

No excuses, put in the work.

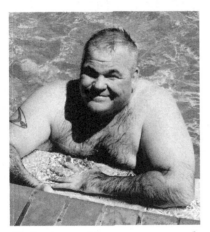

Relaxing with some sun and
water therapy.

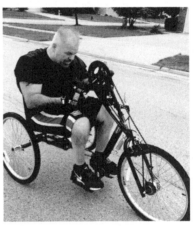

Out for a bike ride.

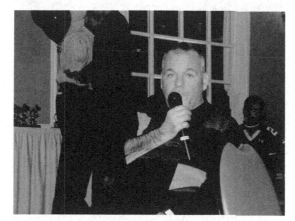
Brian sharing some inspiration.

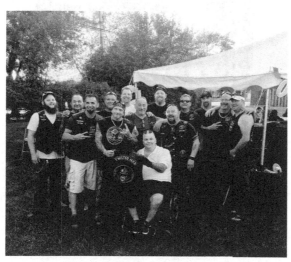
Twisted Aces

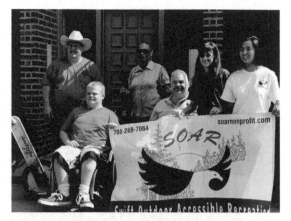

Swift Outdoor Accessible Recreation (SOAR)
finding ways to make the outdoors accessible for those in need.

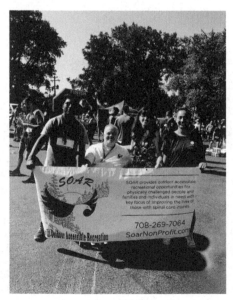

SOAR sponsoring and participating in a triathlon to
support a local veterans home.

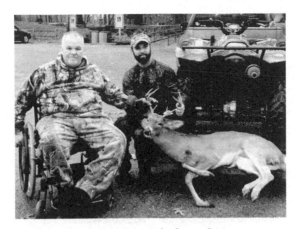

Hunting with friends.

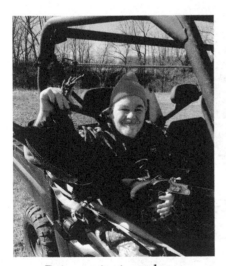

Brian enjoying a hunt.

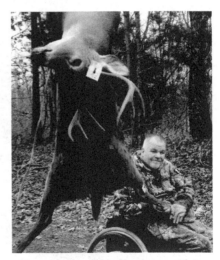

Brian proudly displaying his
trophy 8 point.

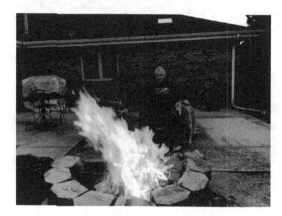

Outdoor fire therapy.

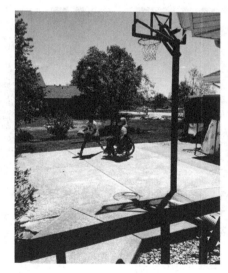

Court time with my son.

1 4

I Don't Have Any Faith

"Every man has but one destiny."
–Mario Puzo, The Godfather

Faith can be defined as confidence in what we hope for and assurance about what we do not see. I believe that faith is essential to blessings and success. I never asked God to help me walk, but I did ask Him to give me the strength and courage to deal with the hand I have been dealt.

Our lives are filled with so many blessings that many times we don't even recognize them. In order for you to have those blessings, you have to be faithful. God allows your faith to be tested in different ways. Allow God to grow your faith, and you will grow as a better person.

I can tell you two irrefutable facts: there is a God, and I am not Him. I would also like to add that over the past thirty-nine years of being a C5/6 quadriplegic, I could not have accomplished all the wonderful things I have been blessed with without my faith and God's guidance.

It is difficult to always have positive thoughts and trust our faith during difficult times in our lives. Our need for faith and prayer is imperative when dealing with a spinal cord injury. Paralysis is just as much a physical challenge as it is a mental challenge. The demands on your body due to your injuries can lead to mental paralysis. You start to think too much, which many times does not lead to anything good. At times like these, many people can give up hope and shut down.

This is the time we need to lean on our faith the most. Faith is powerful and can be used to help heal the deep psychological wounds that spinal cord injuries can cause. I'm not saying that if you believe in God and have faith, He is going to make you walk tomorrow. Once we begin to heal psychologically, faith can be drawn on when we need that little extra boost to get through everyday tasks.

I got my strong faith through both of my parents, but mostly through my mom. I have never met a person with such an amazing faith. She is my rock. I doubt that she has received everything she has asked for, but I do believe she has been given everything she needs.

She is an amazing steward of her Catholic faith, and I am blessed to have that instilled in me. To see what she has dealt with and how steadfast her faith and beliefs are is amazing. Her faith causes her to act on what she hasn't experienced yet, to believe promises in the Bible that haven't been fulfilled yet, and to trust God when our situations haven't changed yet.

If you're struggling with your faith, you are not alone. Talk is cheap, and a lot of people talk the talk, but they don't really trust God. They say they believe in God, but they don't really trust Him when it comes to their finances, health, or job.

You will need faith every day of your life. My faith has given me strength. When I say strength, I don't mean a physical strength to lift up a car. I mean the inner resolve to withstand turmoil.

God is looking for faithful people. God is physically, visibly, actively taking the initiative to look for faithful people that He can bless. Without faith, it is impossible to please yourself or God. Some people are doubters because they see the bad in this world and blame God. Having faith is going beyond that to realize that there are other forces in this world that affect our lives and that there is a reason for everything, even when we don't understand what it is.

Remain hopeful, keep the faith, and let it guide you away from fear and worry and toward peace and joy. Faith is a huge force in our lives. As they say, faith can move mountains. I can say this because I have lived it, and I have seen others power through life's bullshit and obstacles without hesitation by relying on their faith. Your heartfelt faith will be an assurance of your future mental strength, courage, integrity, and optimistic attitude, and even more importantly, your salvation.

When you find yourself questioning your faith or wondering why your prayers haven't been answered, look to this prayer for clarity. It isn't that God isn't listening to your prayers; it's just that sometimes His answer is no, and He has other plans for you.

The Creed for the Disabled

I asked God for Strength, that I might achieve.

I was made weak, that I might learn humbly to obey.

I asked for health, that I might do greater things.

I was given infirmity that I might do better things.

I asked for riches, that I might be happy.

I was given poverty, that I might be wise.

I asked for power, that I might have the praise of men.

I was given weakness, that I might feel the need of God.

I asked for all things, that I might enjoy life.

I was given life, that I might enjoy all things.

I got nothing I asked for but everything I had hoped for.

Almost despite myself, my unspoken prayers were answered.

I am, among men, most richly blessed!

Written by a Confederate soldier in the Civil War

Thoughts from the Quadfather: *I guarantee I would not be writ-*

ing this book or be as blessed as I am without faith. I just don't mean faith in God but also faith in myself and faith in others. Your faith will be tested often and in dramatic ways.

I am not going to preach or try to convince you of anything. Thirty-nine years after breaking my neck, I am still not walking, and my faith is stronger now than ever.

1 5

I Don't Have an Education

"There are things that have to be done and you do them and you
never talk about them. You don't try to justify them. They can't be
justified. You just do them. Then you forget it."
–Mario Puzo, The Godfather

It doesn't matter what you don't have because that is behind
you. That's why the windshield is bigger than the rear-view mirror.
What's in front of you is far more important than what's behind you.

There is nothing stopping you from getting your high school
diploma, associate's degree, bachelor's degree, master's degree, or
doctorate. With technology and the instantaneous access to information, coupled with the availability of online classes, there are no
reasons not to get an education. Also, there are so many foundations
that offer grants for education for the disabled that tuition no longer
has to be a financial hardship. You can also apply for state or federal
aid. With junior colleges being so affordable and offering so many
programs, you need to take the opportunity to better yourself with
additional knowledge and wisdom.

Having an education will also help address some other issues
you are struggling with—like "No one will hire me" or "I don't have
enough money." People with more education have knowledge and
skills to perform higher-level employment roles. Also, from a social
view, it adds substance to your resume as a person.

Let's be honest; now that you are disabled, you're in no position to go into the trades or other manual intensive labor. Also, your need for better health benefits to make your life easier to manage is essential. These benefits are mostly found in higher-level employment requiring more education. Education also improves your organizational and time management skills.

Apart from raising income levels, education has the potential to help individuals gain access to networks that could lead to enhanced social outcomes. Maybe the most important thing that education gives you is self-confidence while keeping your mind busy to focus on the positive things in life.

No one is going to hand you anything, so go earn it. I guarantee you will feel better about yourself and life. Now that you have no excuses, go make a call or get online and make it happen!

Thoughts from the Quadfather: Knowledge is power. Get a degree or certification if you don't have one.

One of the fields that are growing is virtual assistance. Also, more companies are having workers work from home as a contractor because it saves them a lot of expenses.

There are so many opportunities and fields you can work in with a computer and a phone. I recommend you try to find something you like doing and make it happen.

16

Why Do I Succeed?

"You can do more. You can be more."
–Brian P. Swift, The Quadfather

I succeed because I am willing to do the things you are not.

I will fight against the odds.

I will sacrifice. I am not shackled by fear, insecurity or doubt.

I feel those emotions—drink them in and then swallow them away
to the blackness of hell.

I am motivated by accomplishment, not pride.

Pride consumes the weak—kills their heart from within.

If I fall, I will get up.

If I am beaten, I will return.

I will never stop getting better.

I will never give up, ever.

That is why I succeed.

–Author unknown

I don't state these facts to brag. I share this with you to show you
what is possible:

At 17, I broke my neck and became a C5/6 quadriplegic

At 21, I graduated from college

At 24, I graduated from law school

At 24, I got a full-time job

At 27, I got married and bought my first house

At 32, we adopted our first child

At 35, we built our fully accessible home

At 38, we adopted our second child

At 40, we adopted our third child

At 51, I had my first book published

At 53, I started a non-profit called Swift Outdoor Accessible Recreation (SOAR)

I have worked for thirty years full- or part-time

How bad do you want it?

Thoughts from the Quadfather: *You have heard me say it is a journey you cannot make alone. I am blessed, and I could not have succeeded at much without the grace of God, the help of friends, and the support of my family. That being said, even with support, without your own desire, determination, and grit, you cannot build a happy, successful life.*

Knowing the support I have been blessed with, I always felt it was my responsibility to be the most optimistic, fun person to be around. It is your responsibility to be the best person you can be. Control what you can control—your attitude, your zest for life, your ability to impact others through your actions.

17

Don't Quit

"If I can believe in myself that much, nothing else matters."
–Mario Puzo, The Godfather

I have carried this poem in my wallet on a little laminated card since I broke my neck. It has been the inspiration many times that I have needed to continue on when things became very difficult. Thirty-nine years later, I still carry it with me. Every day, I see it as a reminder that even though I may experience some hardships that day, I can never quit. I need the strength from that reminder to remember that I am not a quitter. It just isn't in me. It isn't who I am.

Don't Quit

When things go wrong, as they sometimes will,

When the road you're trudging seems all uphill,

When the funds are low and the debts are high,

And you want to smile, but you have to sigh,

When care is pressing you down a bit,

Rest, if you must, but don't you quit.

Life is queer with its twists and turns,

As every one of us sometimes learns,

And many a failure turns about,

When he might have won had he stuck it out;

Don't give up though the pace seems slow—

You may succeed with another blow.

Often the goal is nearer than,

It seems to a faint and faltering man,

Often the struggler has given up,

When he might have captured the victor's cup,

And he learned too late when the night slipped down,

How close he was to the golden crown.

Success is failure turned inside out—

The silver tint of the clouds of doubt,

And you never can tell how close you are,

It may be near when it seems so far,

So stick to the fight when you're hardest hit—

It's when things seem worst that you must not quit.

–*Author unknown*

Thoughts from the Quadfather: *It's simple; winners don't quit, and quitters don't win. That is a choice, not your circumstance.*

We quit in so many little ways. We all have good intentions, but the road to hell is paved with good intentions and excuses. As the poem above says, rest if you must, but don't you quit. You must find ways to keep your mind, heart, and soul positive and moving forward. Remember, your body will follow.

Surround yourself with people that keep you motivated. I have two great friends who live in other states, and we talk several times a month because when I hang up with them, I feel better, recharged, and ready to attack life. It's not that my problems disappear, but I am mentally in a better place.

You must be honest with yourself when you're looking at making excuses or slacking off when it comes to therapy, exercise, school, work, or life in general. Find a mentor or a friend that keeps you fired up. Never Quit.

18

The Journey of a Quad

"Sometimes you must hurt in order to know, fall in order to grow,
lose in order to gain, because most of life's greatest lessons are
learned through pain."
–Unknown

I believe that the average person could not go through the uncertain difficult days, let alone weeks, months, and years that a quadriplegic or others with disabilities have to go through. As a C5/6 quadriplegic, I have been blessed in so many ways, but it has not come easy or without great sacrifice, blood, sweat, and tears.

As blessed as I have been, my life has not been without devastating hardship, trials, and tribulation. Outside of the daily worries of my catheter leaking, having a bowel accident at work or play, and accessibility, I'm also worried about the obligations to my work and family.

The feelings of inadequacies and emasculation that I have felt due to my disability are too numerous to count. Dealing with this is a journey, not a destination. First, you need to consider what you believe defines a man. I can tell you with 100% certainty that you don't have to be walking to be a man.

Being a man is more mental than it is physical, and you have to deal with this the rest of your life. Also remember, life doesn't revolve around you, and the more you give, the more you get.

Other circumstances and adversities I dealt with through the years, which, as my father says, builds character, are:

I had a manual wheelchair for over thirty-nine years

The ten years I lived at home with my parents, our bathroom was not accessible

I spent over a year, while going to school, with elbow braces on to heal my tendentious

Had several kidney infections during school

I had to drive over an hour to my first job

My wife and I went through five unsuccessful fertility inseminations

I spent over twenty thousand dollars with an adoption agency, only to be told we probably would not be picked by a mother to adopt her child because of my disability

I spent nine months going through an adoption pregnancy, only to have the birth mother change her mind the morning we were going to pick up the baby

I had an ingrown hair that turned into an abscess on my inner thigh that had to be surgically removed and left me bedridden for three months

I went septic from a kidney stone and had a stint put in my kidney

In ten months, I passed over 25 kidney stones

After the first twenty-five years I spent in a manual wheelchair, I developed tendentious, bursitis, and arthritis in my hands, elbows, and shoulders, which I still suffer from today

I live with chronic pain every day

I shattered both femurs sliding out of my chair in my garage, which required me to spend five months in a hospital bed in our family room

The company I helped start and run let me go while I was recovering from my broken legs

I broke my tibia, fibula, and femur falling out of my chair in my van and spent four months in a hospital bed in our family room

I partially tore my rotator cuff.

Thoughts from the Quadfather: *I have been through hell. I have lived in hell, and I have crawled out of hell mentally, physically, and spiritually. I have a master's degree in Knocked Down and a doctorate degree in Rising Up.*

One of the greatest powers we all have is the power to choose. Successful people have several things in common; they make good choices.

You can act or procrastinate, believe or doubt, pray or curse, and succeed or fail. The solution to avoiding future problems is the good choices you will make today.

Going forward, what you do from this moment on is all you can control. If you fail to achieve something, it will not be because you're confined to a wheelchair or because you did not have an education, money, time, or resources.

These things people claim they are missing is not the defining factor. They are cop-outs. People who fail claim it's because of a lack of resources, but in fact, you lacked resourcefulness like commitment, integrity, attitude, passion, resolve, creativity, and determination.

Do you know who you will talk to more than anyone else in your life? YOU! It is what a person thinks of themselves that really determines their fate, and unfortunately, 80% of our thoughts are negative, and 95% are repetitive.

Making our self-talk optimistic, the things we say to ourselves, the things we think in our own mind's eye when we're alone are critical when bringing about genuine action and change.

The practice of positive self-talk is often the process that allows you to discover the obscured optimism, hope, and joy in any given situation.

Watch your thoughts; they become words.

Watch your words; they become actions.
Watch your actions; they become habit.
Watch your habits; they become character.
Watch your character; it becomes your destiny.

–Lao Tzu

19

Resources

One of the best resources I can give you is thirty-nine years of knowledge, experience, and wisdom of living as a quadriplegic. You also have the benefit of the Internet and technology, but ultimately, your happiness, your success is in your hands. Yes, I understand everyone's circumstance is different and unique. Yes, I understand everyone's injury is different and unique.

That being said, we all have the same ability to seek faith and strength from God.

We all have the same ability to challenge and mentally push ourselves beyond the limits of the statistics and prognosis we have been given.

You can live a rewarding, fulfilling life from a wheelchair or with a disability. You can make a difference, but you can't do it alone. You will need physical assistance, support, and divine strength and inspiration. You will need to dig deeper than you ever have to find this GRIT that is in each of us.

At seventeen, I had no idea what I was capable of. All I knew is that I wanted to do things that I did before my accident and that I had to keep moving forward. Moving forward meant continuing my education, playing sports, driving, getting stronger, doing more therapy, dating, and having fun. I challenged myself and pursued my dreams.

I wish you the best. Have great days, and God bless.

1. Byron Riesch Paralysis Foundation
   Scholarships, Research and Individual Grants for those living
   with Paralysis
   P:(262) 547-2083 | URL: bfpf.org
   P.O. Box 1388 Waukesha, WI 53187

2. Dream2Walk
   Financial Assistance to SCI patients
   P:(214) 417-8466 | URL: dream2walk.org
   1904 Webster Drive – Plano, TX 75075

3. Carson Foundation (Canada & U.S.)
   Grants for Individuals (Maximum = $500 Grants x2 a year)
   P:(416) 918-8711 | URL: www.thecarsonfoundation.com
   17090 Regional Road 50 – Palgrave, ON L7E 0L2

4. Be Perfect SCI Foundation
   Provide Grants to Individuals with SCI and TBI
   P:(909) 621-9309
   720 Indigo Court – Pomona, CA 91767

5. Walking with Anthony
   Support SCI Research, SCI Rehab Centers and Grants to Individuals living with SCI
   P: (310) 745-0090 | URL: walkingwithanthony.org
   9903 Santa Monica Blvd. Suite 104 – Beverly Hills, CA 90210

6. Will2Walk
   Grants Awarded Twice Yearly to Individuals with SCIs
   P:(602) 741-6012 | URL: will2walk.org
   1909 E. Ray Road #9-238 – Chandler, AZ 85225

7. Wheel to Walk
   Serves Athletes Under the Age of 20
   P:(503) 257-1401 | URL: wheeltowalk.com
   PO Box 20146 – Portland, OR 97294

8. Athletes Helping Athletes

Serves Youth Athletes Under Age 18
P:(888) 566-5211 | URL: roadrunnersports.com
5549 Copley Drive – San Diego, CA 92111

9. I'm Able Foundation
Primarily Serves Mid-Atlantic Area
P:(8777) 595-3505 (Extension 4) | URL: imablefoundation.org
220 North Park Rd. – Wyomissing, PA 19610

10. Road to Recovery
Motocross Athletes who suffer a life-altering injury
P:(760) 436-1366 | URL: road2recovery.com
1041 N El Camino Real, Suite B-350, Encinitas, CA 92024

11. Fallen Riders Foundation
Motocross Athletes who suffer a life-altering injury
P:(318) 609-4724 | URL: www.fallenridersfoundation.net/
PO Box 4822, Pineville, LA 71361

12. Tighten the Drag Foundation
Therapy Needs, Specialized Equipment
P:(813) 743-2827
URL: tightenthedragfoundation.org
1630 Carr Street – Lakewood, CO 80214

13. Chanda Plan Foundation
Integrative Therapies for Physical disabilities
P:(303) 246-4290 | P (Alt.): (800) 766-4255
URL: iamtheplan.org
1630 Carr Street – Lakewood, CO 80214

14. Courage Kenney Foundation/Allina Health
Maximizing the quality of life for people of all ages and abilities
by delivering comprehensive, person-centered rehabilitation
throughout life.
P: (612) 775-2589 | E: CKFoundation@allina.com
URL: allinahealth.org
1630 Carr Street – Lakewood, CO 80214

15. Falling Forward Foundation
We make it possible for people to recover from catastrophic medical events.
P: (785) 550-8129 | URL: fallingforward.org
4513 Goldfield – Lawrence, KS 66049DAPTIVE EQUIPMENT

16. Challenged Athletes Foundation (CAF)
Provides funds to be used toward adaptive equipment for those suffering life-altering injury.
P: (858) 866-0959 | URL: challengedathletes.org
9591 Waples Street, San Diego, CA 92121

17. Kelly Brush Foundation
Spring and Fall Equipment Grants for Individuals with Documented Paralysis
P: (802) 846-5298 | URL: kellybrushfoundation.org
3 Main Street, Suite 104 – Burlington, VT 05401

18. SCORE (Spinal Cord Opportunities for Rehabilitation)
Young Athletes, Quality of Life w/ SCI, Medical Care, Home Amenities, Transportation
P: (323) 655-8298 | URL: www.scorefund.org
30 Monument Square Suite 220 – Concord, MA 01742

19. Triumph Foundation
New, Used and Needed Adaptive Equipment
P: (661) 803-3700 | URL: www.triumph-foundation.org
17186 Hickory Ridge Court – Santa Clarita, CA 91387EDICAL EQUIPMENT

20. Travis Roy Foundation
Adaptive Equipment Grants
P: (617) 619-8257 | URL: travisroyfoundation.org
75 State Street, 8th Floor – Boston, MA 02109

21. Friends of Man
Mobility Equipment, Medical Equipment
P: (303) 798-2342 | URL: friendsofman.org

P.O. Box 937 – Littleton, CO 80160

22. Michael-Ryan Pattison Foundation
Support/Fund: Provide Standing Frames and Other Medical
Equipment
P: (425) 466-3030 | URL: acureiscoming.org
15600 NE 8th St. Suite B1 #532 – Bellevue, WA 98008

23. Cindy Donald Dreams of Recovery Foundation
Grants for Individuals & Therapeutic Equipment to Promote
Nerve Regeneration and Gain Muscle Mass
P: (770) 675-6565 | URL: dreamsofrecovery.org
2230 Towne Lake Pkwy, Bldg. 200, Ste. 110, Woodstock, GA
30189HICLEODIFICATIONS

24. Blood Brothers Foundation
Grants for Adaptive Vehicle Modifications
P: (303) 822-7469 | URL: bloodbrothersfoundation.org
P.O. Box 217 – Henderson, CO 80640

25. The Mobility Works Foundation
Grants for Adaptive Vehicles & Driving Aids
P: (866) 723-5991 | URL: themobilityworksfoundation.org
4199 Kinross Lakes Parkway Suite 300 – Richfield, OH 44286

26. The Ralph Braun Foundation
Grants for Mobility Transportation Equipment
P: (800) 488-0359 | URL: braunability.com
"BraunAbility" 631 W. 11th Street – Winamac, IN
46006LITARY

27. America's Fund
Military Personnel Injured after 9/11
P: (760) 725-3680 | URL: semperfifund.org
715 Broadway Street – Quantico, VA 22134

28. Catch A Lift Fund
Serves Post-9/11 Combat Wounded Veterans w/Fitness Pro-

grams and In-Home Gym Equipment
P: (855) 496-4838 | URL: catchaliftfund.com
2066 York Road, Suite 205A – Timonium/Lutherville, MD
21093

29. Dare2Tri
Serves Individuals Who Are Active Participants in Dare2tri for
a Minimum of One Season
P: (312) 967-9874 | URL: www.dare2tri.org
516 N. Ogden Ave. #172 – Chicago, IL 60642

30. Hope for the Warriors
Serves Post–9/11 Service Members and Veterans, Their Families
and Families of the Fallen
P: (877) 246-7349 | URL: hopeforthewarriors.org
8003 Forbes Place, Suite 201 – Springfield, VA 22151

31. Team Possibilities
Grants/Scholarships Awarded to Members of possibilities
P: (909) 558-6384 | URL: teampossabilities.org
8003 Forbes Place, Suite 201 – Springfield, VA 22151

32. The Independence Fund
Serves Military Personnel Only
P: (888) 851-7996 | URL: independencefund.org
9013 Perimeter Woods Drive, Suite E – Charlotte, NC 28216

33. Adaptive Training Foundation
Serves Military Personnel Only
P: (214) 432-1070 | URL: adaptivetrainingfoundation.org/
11837 Judd Ct #120, Dallas, TX 75243

34. Superior Van and Mobility
P: (866) 340-8267 | URL: superiorvan.com
4246 Meghan Beeler Ct., Suite 1, South Bend, IN 46628

35. A–Z MOBILITY
P: (779) 234-9072 | URL: a-zmobility.com
23838 W Industrial Dr N, Plainfield, IL 60585

ADDITIONAL BOOKS
BY BRIAN P. SWIFT

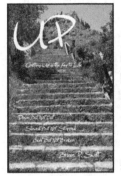

Up Getting Up is the Key to Life

Up Getting Up is the Key to Life is the creation of the author in which he shares his personal paradigm for mental, emotional, and spiritual recovery while facing the challenges of life as a quadriplegic. It is the author's hope to inspire those with similar injuries and give hope to their medical caregivers, family, and loved ones.

Up Getting Up is the Key to Life is the first book by Brian P. Swift. He writes that recovery consists of healing the mind, not just the body and that recovery is a journey, not a destination. The father of three adopted children and husband of over 30 years, Brian developed his strategy of success, CIA: Commitment, Integrity, and Attitude. With his engaging style and practical wisdom, Brian will leave you invigorated to face your own struggles with hope, faith, and purpose!

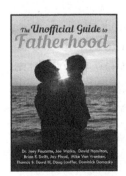

The Unofficial Guide to Fatherhood

The Unofficial Guide to Fatherhood: What makes a band of nine fathers want to write a book on fatherhood? They felt a need to share their struggles and successes. In a melody of stories, advice, and experiences, the authors take you on a journey of men who don't hold back their honesty or enthusiasm about being a proud father. You will find moments of joy, sadness, and triumph. Whether you are a father, a mother, son, daughter, or caregiver, there is something in the book for you. It will kindle your excitement to send a message of love.

Go Ask Your Dad

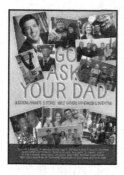

Go Ask Your Dad: A generation of children have heard "Go ask your dad." A culmination of dads from around the country address questions like, How do you raise a daughter? and How do you cope with divorce? to topics like bullying, social-media, forces of terrorism and being a disabled parent. The authors don't claim to be perfect. They do promise, in the book, you will find valuable lessons from their mistakes and successes.

Godly Men Make Godly Fathers

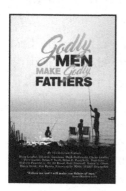

In the pages of Godly Men Make Godly Fathers, you will meet fathers from diverse upbringings and family structures. You will meet men who have endured significant tests to their faith through tragedy and others who have experienced great triumphs. These fathers will take you on a heartfelt journey. Each chapter tackles a unique viewpoint and is written with unconditional faith and love.

A collection of fathers from across the globe share and implement lessons they learned through their Christian faith to encourage fathers, sons, and families. In this book, these men share their Christian values in hopes of spreading the message of joy, love, and family that transcends race, cultures, and generations.

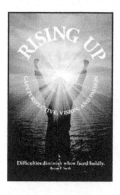

Rising Up

Rising Up is a new book created by author Brian P. Swift in which he shares his personal paradigm for mental, emotional, and spiritual grit and facing the challenges of life as a quadriplegic. Mr. Swift will inspire others as he shares his unique life experience that will equip you with valuable tools to help you overcome adversity and improve your own courage, self-confidence, and grit.

Rising Up will:

- Empower you to get past your own limiting beliefs and challenge your thinking, giving you a different perspective on life.

- Drive you to tap into courage, strength, passion, and the necessary confidence to overcome any challenge, obstacle, and unexpected change that life throws at you.

- Help you create the right mindset to implement success while you create an intentional and purposeful life.

All books can be purchased through Amazon.com, brianpswift. com, or soarnonprofit.com.

NOTES

Chapter 1: Quote from The Godfather March 24, 1972 (USA). Director: Francis Ford Coppola

What Makes A Dad. Author unknown

Chapter 2: Quote from The Godfather March 24, 1972 (USA). Director: Francis Ford Coppola

Swift, Brian P. UP Getting Up is the Key to Life. Mother's House Publishing, 2013

Chapter 3: Quote from The Godfather March 24, 1972 (USA). Director: Francis Ford Coppola

Chapter 4: Quote from The Godfather March 24, 1972 (USA). Director: Francis Ford Coppola

Chapter 5: Quote from The Godfather March 24, 1972 (USA). Director: Francis Ford Coppola

Louv, Richard. Last Child in the Woods: Saving Our Children from Nature-Deficit Disorder. Chapel Hill: Algonquin Press, 2005

Chapter 7: Quote from The Godfather March 24, 1972 (USA). Director: Francis Ford Coppola

www.news.utexas.edu/2014/05/16/mcraven-urges-graduates-   to-find-courage-to-change-the-world, 2016

Swift, Brian P. Rising Up. Motivation Champs Publishing, 2018

Chapter 8: Quote from The Godfather March 24, 1972 (USA). Director: Francis Ford Coppola

Styx. "The Grand Illusion." The Grand Illusion, Paragon Recording Studios, Illinois, 7 July 1977.

Chapter 9: Quote from The Godfather March 24, 1972 (USA). Director: Francis Ford Coppola

Ricotti, Sonia. PassItOn.com, 2018

Chapter 10: Quote from The Godfather March 24, 1972 (USA). Director: Francis Ford Coppola

Chapter 11: Quote from The Godfather March 24, 1972 (USA). Director: Francis Ford Coppola

Swift, Brian P. UP Getting Up is the Key to Life. Mother's House Publishing, 2013

Chapter 13: Quote from The Godfather March 24, 1972 (USA). Director: Francis Ford Coppola

Chapter 14: Quote from The Godfather March 24, 1972 (USA). Director: Francis Ford Coppola

The Creed for the Disabled. Author unknown

Chapter 15: Quote from The Godfather March 24, 1972 (USA). Director: Francis Ford Coppola

Chapter 16: Why Do I Succeed? Source: gotbyouthblog.tumblr.com via Hilary

Chapter 17: Quote from The Godfather March 24, 1972 (USA). Director: Francis Ford Coppola

Don't Quit. Author unknown

Chapter 18: Tzu, Lau. www.goodreads.com. "Watch your thoughts; they become words. Watch your words; they become actions. Watch your actions; they become habit. Watch your habits; they become character. Watch your character; it becomes your destiny" (2018).

The Quadfather

Brian P. Swift

Made in the USA
Middletown, DE
25 May 2021